Studying & Test Taking

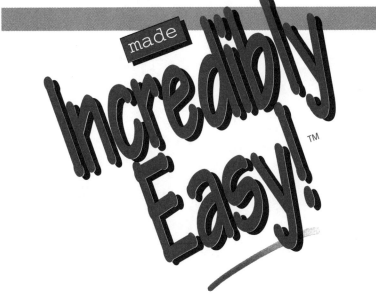

made Incredibly Easy!™

Studying & Test Taking

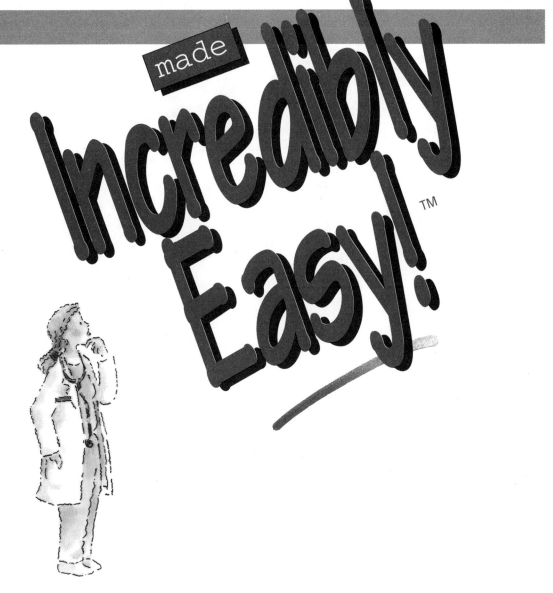

made Incredibly Easy!™

Springhouse Corporation
Springhouse, Pennsylvania

Staff

Vice President
Matthew Cahill

Clinical Director
Judith A. Schilling McCann, RN, MSN

Art Director
John Hubbard

Executive Editor
Michael Shaw

Managing Editor
Andrew T. McPhee, RN, BSN

Clinical Editors
Collette Hendler, RN, CCRN; Joan M. Robinson, RN, MSN, CCRN; Gwynn Sinkinson, RN,C, MSN, CRNP; Beverly Tscheschlog, RN

Editors
Kevin Haworth, Patricia Nale, Patricia Wittig

Copy Editors
Brenna H. Mayer (manager), Virginia Baskerville, Mary T. Durkin, Kathryn Marino, Jaime Stockslager, Pamela Wingrod

Designers
Arlene Putterman (associate art director), Mary Ludwicki (book designer), Joseph John Clark, Jacalyn B. Facciolo

Illustrator
Bot Roda

Typography
Diane Paluba (manager), Joyce Rossi Biletz, Valerie Molettiere

Manufacturing
Deborah Meiris (director), Patricia K. Dorshaw (manager), Otto Mezei (book production manager)

Editorial Assistants
Beverly Lane, Marcia Mills, Liz Schaeffer

Indexer
Barbara Hodgson

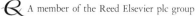 A member of the Reed Elsevier plc group

Library of Congress Cataloging-in Publication Data

Studying and test taking made incredibly easy.
   p. cm.
   Includes index.
   1. Test-taking strategy. 2. Study skills.
   3. Nursing. I. Springhouse Corporation.

DNLM/DLC   99-037384
ISBN 0-58255-019-0 (alk. paper)   CIP

Contents

Contributors and consultants

Lillian Agnes Clary, BA, MA
Associate Dean
Learning Resources
Allan Hancock College
Santa Maria, Calif.

Athena A. Foreman, RN, MSN
Nursing Coordinator
Stanly Community College
Albemarle, N.C.

Joseph W. Slap, MD
Clinical Professor
Thomas Jefferson Medical School
Philadelphia
Training and Supervising Analyst
Philadelphia Association for Psychoanalysis

Rebekah E. Smith, PhD
Postdoctoral Research Fellow
School of Psychology
Georgia Institute of Technology
Atlanta

Diana M. Wagner, BA, MA
Former Director
Learning Enhancement Center
Beaver College
Glenside, Pa.
Advising Coordinator
Seidel School of Education
Salisbury (Md.) State University

Foreword

When facing an examination in a difficult course, do you stride into the testing room, ready to answer any question that comes your way? Do you look forward to writing essays that will allow you to demonstrate your command of the content? Are you fully confident that no matter what questions the instructor asks, you'll know the answer?

Unless you can answer *yes* to all three questions for every course you take, this book is for you. *Studying & Test Taking Made Incredibly Easy* offers a unique approach to make your studying and test-taking skills the best they can be. Filled with tips and strategies, the book covers the learning process, how to maintain the right attitude and motivate yourself to succeed, how to overcome obstacles, how to manage your time more effectively, what steps you can take to improve your reading and note-taking skills, how to prepare for tests, and how to handle math anxiety and reduce stress. It also offers test-taking tips and explains the role of computers and the Internet as learning tools.

Studying & Test Taking Made Incredibly Easy provides just the guidance you need to radically improve your studying and test-taking skills. And it does so in a lighthearted, down-to-earth way. The book is bursting with easy-to-understand strategies sweetened with warmth and humor.

Each chapter is designed to lighten your learning load, not load you down with heavy-handed jargon. You'll learn:
• the importance of having a positive attitude about yourself and your capabilities
• how to set and achieve goals
• ways to improve your concentration and memory and the difference between memory and understanding
• ways to hone your time-management skills, including how to handle procrastination
• how to get the most out of your notes and the classroom experience.

It's never too early to examine chapter 8, which offers tons of tips and strategies for taking all kinds of tests, including:
• essays
• math
• multiple-choice
• oral

- reading comprehension
- short-answer and completion
- true-false
- vocabulary.

In each chapter, you'll find special features designed to enhance understanding and make learning enjoyable. Every chapter begins with an at-a-glance summary of key topics. Self-assessment checklists make it easy to spot important points. A *Quick quiz* at the end of each chapter helps you assess what you've learned.

Special logos throughout the book alert you to essential information. *Advice from the experts* offers time-tested tips and strategies for overcoming specific studying and test-taking obstacles. *Exercise your mind* outlines activities you can use to improve your studying and test-taking skills.

To top it all off, a special section called *Overcoming obstacles* answers all the questions students like you would be most likely to ask about difficult studying and test-taking issues. For instance, this section answers such questions as, "How do I avoid procrastinating?" "How can I stop myself from becoming so anxious before a test?" and "What can I do if a test question completely stumps me?"

I know that, after you check out this useful and refreshingly original book, you'll agree that *Studying & Test Taking Made Incredibly Easy* is the most enlightening and enjoyable study reference ever. With this unique resource by your side, you'll feel more confident and well-prepared than ever before.

Come on, bring on those tests!

Lillian Agnes Clary, BA, MA
Associate Dean
Learning Resources
Allan Hancock College
Santa Maria, Calif.

Part I Learning

The learning process

Just the facts

In this chapter, you'll learn:

♦ how the brain controls reason, thinking, movement, sensory perception, emotions, and all vital functions

♦ why learning increases the number of synaptic connections made between neurons

♦ how the cerebral cortex controls the brain's highest-level functions, such as sight, hearing, memory, and thought

♦ why left-brained people tend to be linear thinkers, and right-brained people tend to be more visually oriented

♦ why food plays an integral role in helping the brain carry out its functions effectively

♦ why each person has a different style of learning; some are visual learners, and others are more hands-on learners

♦ what critical thinking is and how it's used to process information.

All about the brain

The human brain, a complex, 3-lb (1.35-kg) mass of nerve tissue, is an elaborate extension of the spinal cord. All learning takes place in the brain. Understanding the brain can help you become a more successful learner. This chapter examines basic facts about the brain and how it works and then delves into the physiologic mechanisms of learning.

Functions

A popular notion exists that in most people only a fraction of the brain's capacity is used. That notion, for all of its ramifications, is accurate. Moreover, a person would be hard-pressed to make even close to full use of the brain's astounding potential.

The brain performs a number of critical functions, among them:
• controlling the body's involuntary functions, such as breathing, circulation, and temperature regulation
• making voluntary actions possible
• controlling emotional reactions
• maintaining balance and equilibrium
• allowing a person to interpret sensory information that arrives through the eyes, ears, and other sense organs
• regulating reasoning and thinking.

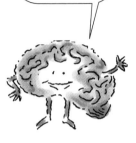

I think the brain is the mightiest organ in the body. Of course, that's just me.

Areas of the brain

Each area of the brain performs certain functions. The brain is composed of three major areas:
• brain stem
• cerebellum
• cerebrum. (See *Brain anatomy.*)

Multifaceted brain stem

The brain stem houses cell bodies for most of the cranial nerves and includes the midbrain, pons, and medulla oblongata. The midbrain controls pupillary reflexes and eye movements. The pons helps regulate respirations and controls chewing, taste, saliva secretion, hearing, and equilibrium. The medulla oblongata influences cardiac, respiratory, and vasomotor functions.

Excitable reticular activating system

A diffuse network of hyperexcitable neurons, the reticular activating system (RAS) fans out from the brain stem through the cerebral cortex. After screening all incoming sensory information, the RAS channels it to appropriate areas of the brain for interpretation.

Multitasking midbrain

The midbrain links the brain stem to the thalamus (for information relay) and to the hypothalamus (instrumental in

Brain anatomy

Many areas of the brain are involved with learning and retention. This diagram reviews major areas of the brain.

Cerebral cortex

Temporal lobe
Cerebellum
Brain stem

Frontal lobe

regulating drives and actions). The hypothalamus is an integral part of the limbic system, which lies above the brain stem and consists of a number of interconnected structures. Researchers have linked these structures to hormones, drives, temperature control, emotion, and memory formation. The hippocampus, part of the midbrain, plays a crucial role in processing various forms of information as part of long-term memory. Damage to the hippocampus can produce global retrograde amnesia or the inability to lay down new stores of information.

The cerebellum, the second largest brain region, lies below the posterior portion of the cerebrum and controls balance and coordination.

Cerebral cerebrum

The cerebrum consists of two hemispheres, the right and left. The highly convoluted surface of the hemispheres — the cerebral cortex — is about 0.078″ (2 mm) thick and has a total surface area of about 1.8 square yards (1.5 m²), about the size of a desktop.

Brain functions

Although interrelated, each area of the brain controls different major functions and processes in the body. The lower portion — the brain stem and cerebellum — mainly control complex basic functions, such as maintaining muscle tone and regulating involuntary actions. The cerebrum contains the largest and perhaps most amazing feature of the human brain — the cerebral cortex.

The cortex is tops

The cerebral cortex, composed of gray matter, is an exceedingly complex structure. It's here that most of the mind's high-level functions — such as sight — are controlled. The cortex also helps coordinate voluntary muscle movements.

One team with two sides

The cortex of the brain is made up of two symmetrical, many-folded sections — the left and right hemispheres. These two hemispheres are involved in two types of thought processes. (See *Left- and right-brain thinking.*) The left hemisphere, which manages movement of the right side of the body, controls language and logical thinking. The right hemisphere, which manages movement on the left side of the body, controls nonverbal processes. Although the two hemispheres of the brain are active all the time, the left hemisphere dominates the conscious thought processes in about 90% of people.

Lobes left and right

Each hemisphere of the brain is divided into four major lobes:
• occipital lobe, which is located at the back of the head and is involved in gathering and interpreting visual input
• parietal lobe, which straddles the center of the cortex and receives sensory stimuli from the entire body (This lobe interprets and integrates sensations, including pain, temperature, and touch. It also interprets size, shape, distance, and texture. The parietal lobe of the nondominant hemisphere is especially important for awareness of body shape.)
• frontal lobe, which controls the brain's responses to input from the body (The frontal lobe is heavily involved in abstract reasoning, decision making, judgment, and lan-

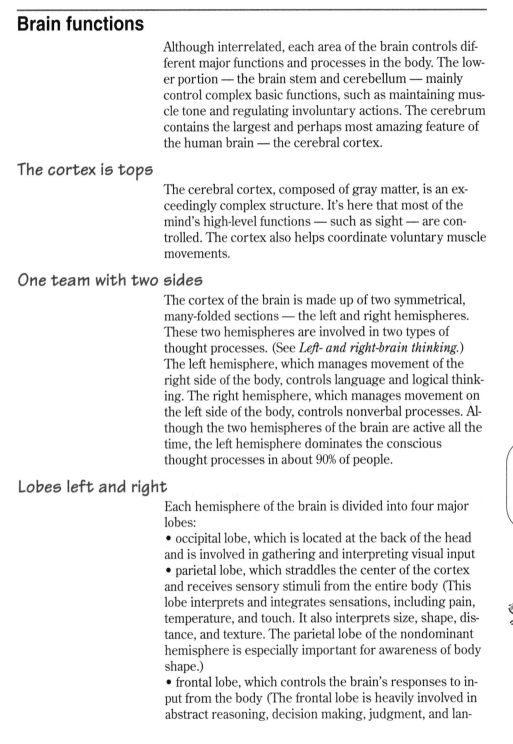

My two hemispheres are further divided into four major lobes.

Now I get it!

Left- and right-brain thinking

Many people think that a person with chiefly pragmatic concerns can be described as being "left-brained," meaning that the left hemisphere is dominant and that a "right-brained" person is more likely to be a free-spirited musician or artist. In reality, despite a person's dominant way of thinking, both sides of the brain are capable and available for skill enhancement. This chart highlights thinking and reasoning tasks for each hemisphere.

Hemisphere	Reasoning tasks
Left	Language and word use
	Logic, reasoning, and analysis
	Numbers and math
	Rational thinking
	Sequences and order
Right	Artistic perception
	Creativity
	Intuitive thinking
	Music and rhythm
	Imagination and abstraction
	Daydreaming and reflection
	Random thinking

guage expression as well as social behavior and movement.)

• temporal lobe, which controls hearing, language comprehension, and storage and recall of memories. (Keep in mind, though, that memories are stored throughout the entire brain.)

Brain cells

The brain is composed primarily of two kinds of cells — glial cells and neurons. Glial cells serve as supporting structures for the brain. Neurons are highly specialized conductor cells that receive and transmit electrochemical nerve impulses. These cells are involved in learning, motion, sensations, and all other complex functions.

Nervous system intersections

Neurons are connected to one another by an extensive network of structures called dendrites and axons. Electrical signals passing through an axon travel at a speed of about 200 miles per hour (100 meters per second).

When the pulse reaches the end of the axon, it causes the release of chemicals called neurotransmitters. These chemicals cross the synaptic gap (a distance of some one-hundredth of a micron) and are picked up by special receptors on the ends of the dendrites of a neighboring neuron. The absorption of the neurotransmitters in this neuron alters the neuron's electrical state and generates a new electrical pulse.

Neuronal connections and learning

Although each person is born with a complete set of neurons, the connections between them are determined largely by learning. External stimuli from sensory cells lead to the development of patterns of nerve impulses, which can alter the strength of the coupling between neurons.

The more often a set of neurons fires together, the stronger the connection between the neurons. The stronger the connection, the more likely that one neuron can more easily stimulate the other neuron to fire when the same external stimulus appears. That's basically what learning is: the neurons "learning" through repetition.

Hormones make for stronger connections

The strength of a connection between neurons relates in large part to the amount of neurohormones available at the synapse. These hormones — such as dopamine, serotonin, and norepinephrine — are crucial in determining the size of electrical signals that pass between neurons. The larger the impulse, the stronger the connection.

Not much rest for the neuro-weary

It takes one-thousandth of a second for a neuron to return to its normal state after passing an impulse along. That means that the neuron can't process another incoming signal for at least that long. In comparison, a modest home computer can process one operation every hundred-millionth of a second or faster!

Rewiring all the time

If a neuron dies, the brain automatically rewires itself to create new connections that go around the dead neuron. Because we lose about 20% of our original neurons during our lifetime, the brain is constantly rewiring itself.

Use it or lose it

Whenever you learn something, the number of connections among the neurons in your brain actually increases. The reverse is true as well: When you stop learning new things, you lose connections that you had before. Through learning, you can rebuild lost connections in the brain, regaining knowledge previously lost and creating more pathways to help you process new information.

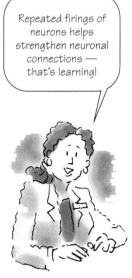

Repeated firings of neurons helps strengthen neuronal connections — that's learning!

Mind-body connection

Keeping the body healthy allows you to learn more efficiently. Begin by keeping your brain in peak running order. Maintain a well-balanced diet and a healthy balance of fluids and electrolytes, substances critical for conducting electrical impulses. Levels of electrolytes such as potassium, chloride, and sodium can enhance or hinder thought processes.

Food for thought

Mood, behavior, and mental performance are influenced by diet, just as physical function is. (See *Brain food,* pages 10 and 11.) To keep mental performance in peak shape, be sure your brain receives the following nutrients:
• amino acids to repair and replace tissues, neurons, and chemicals in the brain
• glucose for energy
• vitamins and minerals to keep neurotransmitter activity healthy.

Eat right

Getting adequate nutrients is easy if you follow a few general dietary guidelines:

Brain food

A number of nutrients affect mental function. This chart highlights key nutrients, their effects on mental function when the diet is deficient in the nutrient, and main food sources of each nutrient.

Nutrient	Effect of deficiency	Source
Vitamins		
B$_1$ (thiamine)	Deficiency can cause confusion, depression, fatigue, or memory loss. Severe deficiency can cause irreversible brain damage or beriberi.	• Beans (legumes) • Brewer's yeast • Pork, fish, and shellfish • Wheat germ and whole grains
B$_2$ (riboflavin)	Deficiency in children can retard brain growth; in adults, it can contribute to behavior problems, depression, and lethargy.	• Almonds • Dairy products • Fruits and green leafy vegetables • Grains, including wheat germ • Poultry
B$_6$ (pyridoxine)	Low levels can worsen premenstrual tension or cause depression or other nervous disorders, irritability, or fatigue due to poor production of serotonin, a neurohormone that promotes relaxation.	• Chicken and seafood • Fruits and vegetables • Peanuts and soy products • Oats, whole grains, and fortified cereals
B$_{12}$ (cobalamin)	Deficiency can contribute to bipolar disorder, chronic fatigue, confusion, insomnia, irritability, memory loss, paranoia, phobias, and restlessness.	• Eggs and dairy products • Fish, red meats, and organ meats
C	Deficiency can cause scurvy and lead to anxiety, depression, excitability, fatigue, or hysteria.	• Citrus and other fruits • Dark green vegetables
Folate (folic acid)	Deficiency can cause depression or lethargy.	• Beans • Brewer's yeast • Green leafy vegetables • Liver • Mushrooms and rice • Wheat germ
Niacin	Minor deficiency can cause anxiety, depression, fatigue, or memory loss. Chronically low levels can lead to pellagra or confusion, hallucinations, or other nervous disorders.	• Brewer's yeast • Legumes and peanuts • Meats, poultry, and seafood • Sunflower seeds

Brain food *(continued)*

Nutrient	Effect of deficiency	Source
Minerals		
Calcium	Short-term deficiency can cause tremors or confusion.	• Sardines and canned salmon • Low-fat dairy products • Kale, soybeans, and tofu • Supplements and some antacids
Iron	Deficiency can lead to difficulties in learning or comprehending.	• Clams, lean meats, and organ meats • Legumes (beans) • Processed tomatoes • Raisins
Magnesium	Low levels in the brain can cause agitation, confusion, depression, irritability, or tremors.	• Green leafy vegetables • Meats, seafood, and soy tofu • Milk and dairy products • Nuts • Sunflower seeds • Wheat germ
Zinc	Low levels in the brain can impair memory. Severe deficiency can cause depression, lethargy, or irritability. Long-term deficiency can cause aggression, disinterest, hyperactivity, mental retardation, or dyslexia.	• Beef, poultry, fish, and shellfish • Grains, wheat bran, and wheat germ

• Eat a variety of foods every day, including vegetables, fruits, grains, and low-fat protein sources.

• Choose low-fat foods, especially those low in saturated fat and cholesterol.

• Use sugars, salts, and vegetable oils in moderation.

• Drink plenty of (nonalcoholic) fluids.

• Achieve and maintain a healthy weight by balancing your caloric intake and energy expenditure.

The pasta connection

No single food can boost your brain power, but high-carbohydrate foods such as pasta can help improve your mood and put you in the best state of mind for learning. Car-

May I suggest a well-balanced diet por vous, to help you study smart?

bohydrates are easily converted to glucose, a simple sugar that provides energy to the brain. Glucose in turn triggers the production of serotonin, a chemical that strongly affects mood and emotion.

Serotonin helps you stay calm and relaxed and can improve your ability to concentrate. It also aids sleep and reduces anxiety in stressful situations. The delicious conclusion: Eating spaghetti can help you improve your studying skills.

Regardless of what you eat, watch the size of the portions. Consuming too many calories at once can make you sleepy, and you can't study when you're sleepy.

Learning styles

There are a number of different learning styles, including visual, auditory, kinesthetic, global, and detail learning. Everyone prefers one or more of these learning styles. To improve your studying and test-taking skills, draw on your preferred style to maximize learning. But don't neglect the other styles either. Becoming a flexible learner using a number of different learning styles can help increase your interest in courses and improve your chances for success.

Seeing is believing

If you learn best by watching how something is done or by reading about it, you're a visual learner. To make the most of this learning style, take advantage of all the visual information available to you, including such written and graphic information as:
- books
- demonstrations
- handouts
- Internet resources
- personal notes
- periodicals
- videos.

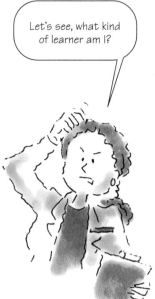

Let's see, what kind of learner am I?

Sounds like...

If you tune in best to things you hear, you're an auditory learner. To make the most of this learning style, use all the auditory information available to you, including:
- discussion with others
- lectures

- question-and-answer sessions
- reading or reciting procedures aloud
- study groups
- tape recordings.

Can do

If you prefer to jump right in and do something new and if your motto could be "Learn by doing," you're a kinesthetic learner. To make the most of your preferred learning style, take every opportunity to:
- attend workshops
- give return demonstrations
- go on field trips
- participate in individual and group projects
- take part in special or extracurricular activities
- tutor others
- volunteer in the classroom or in some area pertinent to the topic.

The big picture

If you find you're always looking at the big picture, chances are you're a global learner. Sweeping theories and overall trends fill your vision. You may perform best when instructed by a teacher who uses analogies and stories or who talks frequently about how things are interrelated. You're most likely to thrive in a classroom where the instructor draws information out by giving hints and leading students to reach conclusions after considering all the angles.

If you're a big picture kind of person, you're probably a global learner.

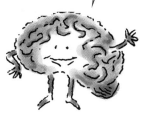

To make the most of your global learning style:
- write summaries of your class notes
- use diagrams to show how small pieces of information relate to the big picture
- develop question lists about the topics you're studying.

Learning is in the details

If you're concerned about following instructions closely and proceeding in a logical order, you're probably a detail learner. You're most comfortable with a teacher who closely follows an outline or lesson plan. Your classroom notes are probably organized from top to bottom, listing broader theories followed by lists of supporting details. You probably believe that in gaining knowledge, conducting impeccable research is as important as reaching a conclusion.

To make the most of detail learning:
- created bulleted summary lists from your class notes
- use diagrams to connect specific ideas to larger concepts
- make specific to-do lists before beginning a study session
- write questions as they occur to you when reading
- be prepared to illustrate specific details with examples.

Learning process

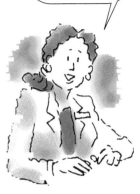

Bloom's learning levels help us understand how we learn, so we can learn more effectively.

Cognitive learning is a process that takes place in stages. A psychologist named Benjamin Bloom described these stages in 1956: knowledge, comprehension, application, analysis, synthesis, and evaluation. (See *Bloom's learning levels.*) Other theories about cognitive learning have since evolved. In these theories, the stages might have different names or occur in a somewhat different progression, but the stages originally described by Bloom remain essentially intact.

A little knowledge

The knowledge stage of critical thinking requires little more than minor memorization skills for recounting information verbatim. It requires little in the way of complex understanding. Examples of information that you may need to recall include:
- mathematic formulas
- names, addresses, phone numbers
- product brand and generic names
- simple instructions.

The meaning of comprehension

The comprehension stage of critical thinking involves converting information from the form in which you receive it to your own words. Many examples of translation can be found in notes you might take as you gather information. Examples of comprehension include:
- making illustrations and diagrams
- paraphrasing
- using shorthand notations and symbols
- writing summaries
- describing cause-and-effect
- describing relationships
- explaining a concept to someone else.

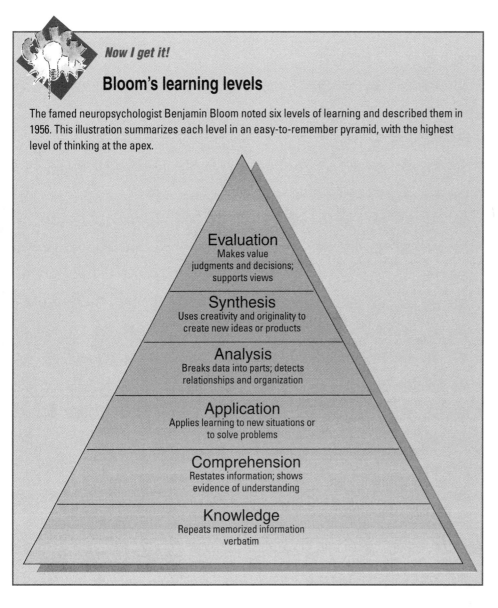

Now I get it!

Bloom's learning levels

The famed neuropsychologist Benjamin Bloom noted six levels of learning and described them in 1956. This illustration summarizes each level in an easy-to-remember pyramid, with the highest level of thinking at the apex.

Evaluation
Makes value judgments and decisions; supports views

Synthesis
Uses creativity and originality to create new ideas or products

Analysis
Breaks data into parts; detects relationships and organization

Application
Applies learning to new situations or to solve problems

Comprehension
Restates information; shows evidence of understanding

Knowledge
Repeats memorized information verbatim

Apply here

In the application stage, you apply the information you've gained, translated, and interpreted to solve problems or

accomplish concrete tasks. Examples of the application stage include:
- completing a project by following directions
- grouping or classifying information by using a rule or principle
- solving math and word problems
- using a theory or formula to solve a new problem
- using prior understanding to solve new problems.

Analyze this

In the analysis stage, you can break down a concept into its parts and understand how it works. For example, you understand the parts of the hand so well and how they work that you can visualize or explain what happens when you pick up a pencil. Other examples of the analysis stage include:
- identifying assumptions
- recognizing logical fallacies such as stereotypes
- deciding whether data are relevant or valid
- recognizing organizational structure.

Synthesize that

In the synthesis stage, you can put parts together to form a new or larger whole. At this level, your thinking processes become more creative and complex. Examples of synthesis include:
- developing your research notes into a paper or oral presentation
- developing a plan for a lab experiment
- writing a short story or poem.

Evaluation time

In the evaluation stage of learning, you reach the most complex level of cognitive functioning. In this stage, you use all other stages to determine the value and relevance of information. Examples of evaluation include:
- judging which conclusions are supported by data
- determining the value of writing, art, or music based on internal criteria or established external criteria
- judging the value of information being presented in a lecture or group discussion.

Evaluation is the most complex level of cognitive functioning. It's also the last step in the nursing process. See a connection?

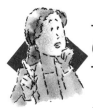

Quick quiz

1. The pons helps control:
    A. heart rate and speech.
    B. respirations and hearing.
    C. digestion and touch.
Answer: B. The pons helps regulate respirations and controls chewing, taste, saliva secretion, hearing, and equilibrium.

2. The left hemisphere controls:
    A. movement on the right side of the body and nonverbal processes.
    B. movement on the left side of the body, language, and logical thinking.
    C. movement on the right side of the body, language, and logical thinking.
Answer: C. The left hemisphere manages movement of the right side of the body and controls language and logical thinking. The right hemisphere manages movement on the left side of the body and controls nonverbal processes.

3. Dopamine, serotonin, norepinephrine, and other neurohormones are crucial in determining the:
    A. size of electrical signals that pass between neurons.
    B. speed at which electrical signals pass between neurons.
    C. duration of activity of electrical signals that pass between neurons.
Answer: A. Dopamine, serotonin, norepinephrine, and other neurohormones are crucial in determining the size of electrical signals that pass between neurons. The larger the impulse, the stronger the connection.

4. According to Bloom's learning levels, the level of learning in which the person breaks data into parts and detects relationships is:
    A. analysis.
    B. application.
    C. synthesis.
Answer: A. Analysis involves breaking data into parts and detecting relationships and organization.

Scoring

☆☆☆   If you answered all four questions correctly, way to go!
You're Benjamin Bloomin' wonderful!

☆☆   If you answered three questions correctly, outstanding!
You're clearly kinesthetically capable!

☆   If you answered fewer than three questions correctly,
don't worry. You're still our favorite synthesizer!

2

Attitude and motivation

Just the facts

In this chapter, you'll learn:

♦ why goals are more likely to be achieved when they're personal rather than set by others

♦ why goals should be specific and have a completion date

♦ how motivation can be intrinsic (personal desire) or extrinsic (physical reward)

♦ why a student with a good attitude should take a positive, responsible approach to a studying task.

Attitude

Attitude is the approach you take to a task. It's often a reflection of how much interest you have in a task or how meaningful the task is to you. Your attitude toward learning, studying, and test taking affects the goals you set for yourself and the techniques and strategies you use to reach those goals. Attitude also strongly affects the level of success achieved in improving your learning skills.

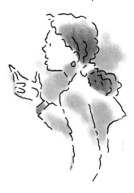

Your attitude about studying directly affects how far you'll travel in your learning.

How attitude affects studying

When you approach a difficult subject with the right attitude, you can:
- gain a clear idea of your role in learning
- establish clear learning goals
- study more efficiently
- achieve better grades and academic performance.

It's up to you

Having the right attitude can be described as having a willingness and desire to learn. Here are attributes of the "right stuff."
• The student accepts responsibility for learning rather than expecting others to teach her.
• The student participates in the learning process rather than being a passive recipient of knowledge.
• The student actively listens, raises questions, and actively seeks answers to those questions.
• The student takes charge of what will be learned from the course and, in effect, how well she'll do in the course.

Got it?

How do you know if you have the right attitude about studying? Find out more about your own attitude by checking the attitude meter. (See *Attitude meter.*)

Developing a winning attitude

A student with a winning attitude expects success, even when tackling the most complex new material. Such students have faith in their own abilities, particularly in their ability to attend classes, complete assigned readings, conduct research, and understand the material presented. Building and using support systems, taking care of yourself, and maintaining consistent focus on your goals are key to having and keeping a winning attitude.

Working together is a winning combination!

A little help, please

One way to build and maintain a winning attitude is to seek out and accept support from other people and resources, including:
• colleagues
• fellow students
• formal and informal discussion groups
• friends and family
• resource centers, such as libraries and media centers
• teachers and tutors.

Exercise your attitude

Attitude is often reflected in how well a person takes care of herself. Getting enough sleep, eating properly, and exercising can help maintain a healthy mind, body, and atti-

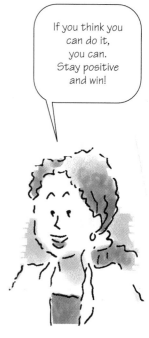

Exercise your mind

Attitude meter

Each of the following statements describes someone with a positive attitude. How many of the traits do *you* have?

- You're naturally good at studying.
- You're strongly interested in learning, regardless of the topic.
- You're receptive to new information.
- You don't rely strictly on a teacher to tell you what to study.
- You have faith in yourself and your ability to learn.
- You use a support system as often as possible.
- You take care of your mind and body.
- You keep a consistently positive attitude.

> If you think you can do it, you can. Stay positive and win!

tude. Looking good and feeling good are big attitude boosters.

Steady as she goes

It's important to keep a positive attitude for the long haul rather than backsliding into complacency in the middle of a task. Developing a good attitude may take time, but it's worth the effort. A consistently positive attitude allows you to cope effectively even in the face of minor setbacks and major disasters.

Motivation

Motivation is the carrot on a stick that inspires the proverbial mule to move forward. It's the thing that makes a person *want* to do something. Motivation:
- causes a person to initiate an activity. In the case of studying, the motivation may be the need for achievement, a high test score, or a good grade.
- helps the person move toward a goal, closing the gap between the starting point and the final objective.
- spurs the person to persist in her attempts to reach the goal until she succeeds.

How motivation affects studying

Motivation to improve study skills and succeed at learning may be intrinsic (an inborn factor that drives a person to learn) or extrinsic (a benefit derived from learning).

Coming from within...

Intrinsic motivation includes:
- a general desire to learn
- a sense of curiosity
- a willingness to take risks
- an innate sense of wanting to excel at something
- an inherent interest in the subject.

...Or without

Extrinsic motivation includes the desire for:
- better grades or test scores
- improved self-esteem
- a sense of fulfillment
- increased competence in the subject
- valuable credentials on a resume
- a better job
- an opportunity to earn a higher salary.

Toward a gold star

Think back to when you were in elementary school. At that time, the reward you might have received for a job well done might have been a gold star. The teacher's idea was to establish that sticker as a motivator, something you would value and strive to earn.

Adults can establish their own sources of motivation. At the start of a task, decide what your reward will be for your hard work. You may decide that the work itself may be its own reward, but you may find it more inspiring to aim for something more — a pat on the back, lunch out with friends, new shoes, or a few days of rest and relaxation.

Choosing a motivator

When choosing a motivator, aim high. Choose a motivator that makes the hard work worthwhile. Then be sure to collect the reward.

Don't underestimate the value of intangible rewards either. You may find that reveling in a sense of satisfaction or accomplishment may be a stronger motivator than

A reward for yourself can help keep you motivated to do your best.

earning a more tangible reward.

Where do motivators come from?

To gain insight into personal motivators, think about things you do on a regular basis and then determine the source of motivation for completing each task. For example, suppose you exercise at a gym twice a week. Why do you do that? To look and feel good? To get your dollar's worth of membership dues? To meet new people?

Identifying and understanding your particular motivating factors for non-school-related situations can help you successfully find motivating factors for school-related situations.

Aim high when choosing a motivator. Then be sure to collect the reward when you succeed.

Long-lasting rewards

A wide range of long-lasting rewards can be gained from developing successful study habits and improving your test-taking skills. Those rewards include:
• ability to apply improved skills to other subject areas
• deeper understanding of the subject matter
• enhanced self-esteem, leading to greater success in other areas of endeavor
• improved grades and test scores
• improved socioeconomic status as a result of learning marketable skills.

Setting goals

Procrastination, poor concentration, and lack of motivation take root when a student lacks clear goals. Without clearly defined goals, it's easy to become distracted. To avoid distraction, set goals for yourself.

Some goals should be easy to reach, some hard, some long-term, and some short-term. The more attractive the goal, the more motivated you'll be. The goal should be specific and include a time for completion. Setting a date for completion of the goal helps you to focus on the goal and gives your day-to-day tasks a sense of purpose.

Accomplishing a goal

Accomplishing a goal involves creating a measurable and achievable goal, determining that the goal is something worth working toward, and devising strategies to achieve the goal.

Make it measurable

A goal should be stated in measurable terms. For example, "I want to master the double-entry system of note-taking by the end of October" is a more specific objective than "I want to improve my study skills."

Make it achievable

Determine whether the goal is achievable. Is there enough time to pursue the goal and, more important, do you have the necessary skills, strengths, and resources to achieve the goal? If not, modify the goal to make it achievable.

Make it desirable

Make certain that achieving the goal is genuinely desirable and worthwhile. The goal should have a positive impact on your life and be consistent with your most important basic values.

In addition, determine why the goal is worthwhile. Make sure that reaching the goal will give you a sense of accomplishment.

Make your goals desirable and achievable.

Create strategies for success

Anticipate potential problems in meeting your goal. In your mind, take yourself step by step through your plan for achieving the goal and ask yourself what can go wrong at each step. Then plan ways to prevent or overcome these problems.

At the same time, devise strategies and steps for achieving the goal. What will you need to begin? What comes next? Then set a timeline for accomplishing each step. (See *Accomplishing a short-term goal.*)

Goal structures

Students in a classroom can be greatly influenced by other people involved in accomplishing the same

Exercise your mind

Accomplishing a short-term goal

Short-term goals can be accomplished by following a series of steps that gradually move you toward your goal. To accomplish a short-term goal:

• Write the goal in measurable terms.

• Set a date for completing the goal.

• Check that the goal is achievable in the time allotted.

• Identify potential problems and determine ways of preventing them.

• Create a series of specific steps for achieving the goal.

• Set a schedule for completion of each step.

goal. The influence of others on your goals has been called the goal structure of the task. Three goal structures have been identified:

• cooperative, in which students believe their goal is attainable only if other students will also reach the same goal

• competitive, in which students believe they will reach their goal only if other students don't

• individualistic, in which students believe their own attempt to reach a goal isn't related to other students' attempts to reach goals.

Grades and goals

If a teacher concentrates class efforts on competitive grading, students tend to focus on performance goals rather than learning goals. Do as much as you can to focus on learning rather than focusing on getting a good grade or doing the work just to get it finished. By understanding the value of the assigned work and how the information you gain will be useful in the future, you can more readily prepare for learning and thus become more successful.

Grades as motivators

That doesn't mean, however, that you shouldn't consider grades at all. Grades are an integral part of the entire school experience and can be powerful motivators themselves. Grades also serve as checkpoints to help you evaluate your progress and adjust your plan for success accordingly. Try to use the desire to earn good grades as a short-term goal without sacrificing the more important long-term goal of getting a good education.

Personal payload

When you're forced to do something you don't really want to do, you'll be less likely to succeed because the goal isn't your own. The successful student must *want* to succeed, and learning itself should be a primary goal.

> To succeed, you must truly *want* to succeed. Go for it!

Reaching your goals

Approach each goal you've set for yourself consistently and with a clear sense of purpose. Reaching your goals involves setting goals continuously, monitoring your progress, determining time frames for your goals, prioritizing goals, challenging yourself to reach higher goals, committing to success, revising your goals when necessary, and linking short-term goals with longer-term ones.

Getting into the goal-setting habit

If you haven't already begun to set goals, start the habit now. If the goals you've identified so far haven't motivated you as well as you had hoped they would, review the goals and, if necessary, set new ones.

Write down your goals

Keep a journal for long-term, intermediate, and short-term goals. Use to-do lists to keep track of the immediate goals that form a part of everyday life. You'll tend to commit your resources more readily to a written goal than to one you've only thought about but haven't recorded. In addition, writing the goal makes the goal more concrete and easier to review periodically.

Divide goals according to a time scale

List goals according to how long it will take to reach them. Typical goal divisions are long-term (5 to 10 years), intermediate (3 to 5 years), short-term (6 months to 2 years), and immediate (this month, this week, or today). Prioritize your goals. Without priorities, you may spend your energy trying to achieve too many goals at once.

Challenge yourself

Keep your goals high enough to inspire you and reasonable enough to seem always within your reach. For example, if your long-term goal is to be a nurse practitioner, your intermediate goal may be to finish nursing school. You may find that your greatest challenge lies in becoming one of the top students in your class.

Commit to success

Commit to the actions required to achieve the goal. Understand that you may not succeed immediately. Learn from your failures and reassess your action plan.

Rewrite, revise, revisit, review

Review your goals and revise them as necessary. At certain points, more inspiring goals may present themselves and short-term and immediate goals may require frequent revision. It's better to change goals and strategies as circumstances change than to lose focus on your long-term goals by refusing to change short-term ones.

Link your goals

Long-term, intermediate, short-term, and immediate goals should be linked in focus to your overriding goals. For example, reading 15 pages of course material today (your immediate goal) leads to achieving a good grade in the class (short-term goal), which leads to graduation from nursing school (intermediate goal), which in turn leads to the opportunity to become a nurse practitioner (long-term goal).

> Goal setting is only a tool. Be sure to enjoy your journey and every success on the way.

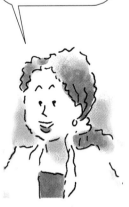

Types of goals

Long-term study goals generally relate to career goals, although some people simply enjoy studying as a means of self-improvement. Again, if the long-term goal is truly the student's choice, then the student is self-motivated and excited about the result, prompting the student to keep studies on track. Like a basketball player who keeps a photo of Michael Jordan on the refrigerator, having some tangible reminder of that long-term goal is useful.

The relay

Intermediate goals are usually 3 to 5 years in the future and are keys to achieving long-term goals. For example, careers that require extended education necessitate the intermediate goal of acceptance into the appropriate centers for higher learning.

Hops, skips, and jumps

The steps toward the intermediate goal are a series of short-term goals, usually set 6 months to 2 years in the future. Particularly when studying toward a goal (a certain degree), the short-term goals could be set per semester or per academic year.

The dash

Each short-term goal can be further divided into smaller tasks, or immediate goals, which can be accomplished in 30 minutes to an hour on a daily basis until each study task is completed. A series of 15 to 20 small tasks might be part of the plan for completing an otherwise frustrating 20-page paper. The result is a finished essay and the chance to experience 15 to 20 successes along the way. (See *Accomplishing a long-term goal.*)

> Keep your eye on your intermediate goals—3 to 5 years away.

Oh, what to do, what to do?

When immediate goals are listed and prioritized, a daily to-do list is created. Each goal must:
- be reasonable (can be done in 30 to 60 minutes)
- be specific
- be verifiable or measurable (can be crossed off the list when it's completed)
- have a payoff (reward) at the end.

Treats for triumph

Rewards give you additional reasons to reach a goal. A reward can be small or large, depending on the person and the goal. To serve as an effective motivator, a reward

Memory jogger

Setting goals is an invitation to success. As with any invitation, you should **RSVP.** Make your goals **r**easonable, **s**pecific, **v**erifiable, and with a **p**ayoff at the end.

Exercise your mind

Accomplishing a long-term goal

Although long-term goals can be daunting to think about, keeping an eye focused on them can help you accomplish short-term goals more successfully. To accomplish a long-term goal, begin by describing where you want to be in 20 years. What do you want to be doing, and where? Write down these 20-year goals. Then ask yourself these questions:

• What will you need to accomplish in 5 years to be able to reach your 20-year goal? Write down these goals as your 5-year goals.

• What will you need to accomplish in 6 months to be able to reach each 5-year goal? Write down these goals as your 6-month goals.

• What will you need to accomplish this week to reach your 6-month goals? Write down these goals as your weekly goals.

Examine the goals
Now list at least five reasons why it's important for you to reach your 20-year goal. List at least three negative things that could happen if you don't reach your goal.

should be desirable. You might reward yourself with dinner at your favorite restaurant or that CD you've had your eye on for the last few weeks.

The reward should also fit the task. That means finishing a task that takes all of 30 minutes doesn't necessarily warrant a weekend shopping trip.

Peers and punishment

Besides rewards, other types of external motivation include peer pressure and punishment. By sharing goals with a friend, you create additional pressure to perform. Punishment, when you deny yourself certain privileges if you don't complete a task, rarely works as a motivator.

Missing the mark

If you fall short of a short-term goal, you may become discouraged and miss a step toward achieving a long-term goal. Try to recoup the loss by reviewing your goals and adjusting them and their deadlines as appropriate. (See *Evaluating a goal,* page 30.) In the long run, it's more efficient to achieve the goal in the first place, even if it's a little behind schedule.

If you miss your goal, try to remain upbeat. Review your goal, and adjust as necessary.

Exercise your mind

Evaluating a goal

Evaluating a goal is a different process than creating one. Evaluation allows you to create more useful, achievable goals. Practice evaluating a goal by completing this exercise. For each goal, decide whether the goal is satisfactory or if it's lacking in some way. Use the key to denote your decision. Keep in mind that if a goal is unsatisfactory, more than one letter may apply.

Key

S — Satisfactory

M — Measurable outcomes lacking

D — Deadline lacking

O — Other people are needed to achieve the goal

Goals

1._____Define my success in each clinical rotation by my score on the first plan of care.

2._____Know all assigned mathematical formulas by the end of next month.

3._____Appreciate art more fully as the result of visiting an art gallery.

4._____By Tuesday, identify the handouts to be used for the final examination.

5._____Learn more about genetic engineering.

6._____Become a better reader.

7._____Improve my Anatomy and Physiology grade by one quality point by participating in a group-study project before the end of the term.

8._____Complete all assigned medical-surgical readings by next Wednesday.

9._____Read my notes immediately following each nutrition class so I can make additions or corrections.

10._____Improve my grade in Fundamentals by 10 points between the mid-term examination and the final examination by joining a study group and meeting with the group 3 days a week for the rest of the marking period.

Your goals

List five of your own goals, and evaluate them.

1._____

2._____

3._____

4._____

5._____

Staying on task

Sometimes it's hard to get started on a project or assignment. The important thing is to take some action, even if it's not as much as you had planned. To get yourself started, break a large project down into manageable parts. Then schedule deadlines for completion of each part. Gaining closure on each part, handling deadlines effectively, avoiding "burnout," and juggling all your other responsibilities efficiently will keep you on the right path toward your goals.

From start to finish

Closure is the positive feeling you receive when you finish a task. One way to obtain closure is to divide a task into manageable goals, list them, and check them off the list as each one is finished. For example, to complete a reading assignment on time, divide the total assignment into smaller assignments by setting a certain number of pages as a goal to be reached each day. Every time you reach one of these small goals, you'll feel a sense of closure that will help propel you toward the next goal.

Dueling deadlines

Several tasks might have the same deadline. Although changing from one task to another may give you a break, changing tasks too often actually wastes time. It slows your momentum on one task and necessitates that you'll have to review tasks that have been put aside when you return to them.

To avoid problems from changing tasks too often, determine how much time you have for the task. If you only have an hour, don't switch tasks; an hour isn't enough time to maintain peak efficiency.

When working on a long-term project that needs to be set aside to complete more immediate tasks, stay organized. To ease the return to the first project, make a list of questions, write notes, identify objectives, and compile references, papers, and other materials pertinent to the task. Then keep all the materials in one place so you can reach them easily and get started more quickly on the task.

Gimme a break!

Burnout results when a student works without breaks. Fatigue, boredom, and stress are signs of burnout. Adding breaks into the work plan helps prevent burnout. Taking a 10-minute break every hour will give your brain a rest and provide a chance for you to relax. A break could be recreational such as taking a walk or work-related such as changing tasks (working on a plan of care and then reading a textbook assignment). Planning for breaks decreases interruptions during prime study time.

Another way to avoid burnout is to leave flexibility in your daily schedule. If you schedule commitments too tightly, you won't complete your goals and achieve closure. This defeats you psychologically because you fail to do what you planned. Give yourself a rest with well-planned breaks.

To avoid burnout, give yourself a break now and then. But stay away from the phone and TV!

The juggling act

Everyone has to manage a wide assortment of life activities: fitness, relationships, chores, finances, hobbies, sports, health, work, and others. Add academics and school activities into the mix and the need for organization becomes clear. Set aside time each day for work as well as for play to make the most of your time.

When you face what seems like too many tasks to complete at once, prioritize each task by writing the tasks on paper and then assigning each with a 1, 2, or 3, with 1 being the most important tasks and 3 being those that can wait. Then concentrate on completing the 1s, then the 2s, and finally the 3s. Prioritizing tasks on paper helps you focus on the most important tasks and gives you a sense of accomplishment that you're moving ahead even if you haven't finished all assigned tasks.

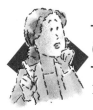

Quick quiz

1. An intrinsic motivator can be defined as:
   A. a benefit derived from learning.
   B. an inborn factor that drives a person to learn.
   C. a learning experience based on attitude or morals.
Answer: B. Motivation may be intrinsic (an inborn factor that drives a person to learn) or extrinsic (a benefit derived from learning).

2. A student with a positive attitude toward studying probably also:
   A. cares about the way she looks and feels.
   B. has more time to complete assignments.
   C. has fewer outside commitments than other students.
Answer: A. The student with a positive attitude toward studying is probably also happy with her personal and physical self.

3. Immediate goals are those that can be accomplished each day in:
   A. 5 to 10 minutes.
   B. 10 to 30 minutes.
   C. 30 minutes to 1 hour.
Answer: C. Each short-term goal can be divided into smaller tasks, or immediate goals, which can be accomplished in 30 minutes to an hour on a daily basis until each study task is completed.

4. Common signs of study burnout include:
   A. fatigue and boredom.
   B. anger and resentment.
   C. denial and depression.
Answer: A. Fatigue, boredom, and stress are signs of burnout. Adding breaks into the work plan helps prevent burnout.

Scoring

☆☆☆   If you answered all four questions correctly, congratulations! You earn an A in Attitude and a week's vacation at the South Sea isle of Intrinsic Motivation!

☆☆   If you answered three questions correctly, way to go! You earn two tickets to the Goalkeepers' Ball!

☆   If you answered fewer than three questions correctly, chin up. A new class in Mastering Motivation starts soon.

Concentration and memory

Just the facts

In this chapter, you'll learn:

♦ how the brain processes through registration, short-term memory, working memory, and long-term memory

♦ why effective study strategies include practice, spaced study, reduction of interference, associations, lists, and imagery

♦ how memory skills can be improved by using various memory enhancement strategies.

Concentration

The more focused your concentration, the more efficiently you can use your study time. To improve your concentration skills, first identify the distractions that impede concentration. Then use one or more study techniques to improve your ability to concentrate and, thus, to learn.

Distractions

Distractions that interfere with concentration can originate from internal or external sources. An internal source is something you think or feel that detracts from focusing on your studies. For example, hunger is an internal source of distraction. So are emotions, such as anger or sadness. External distractions stem from something in your study environment. Loud noises, an uncomfortable chair, or poor lighting are external sources of distraction.

Other distractions

Factors beside internal and external distractions can make concentrating in class or when studying difficult. (See *Meandering mind.*) The instructor may speak rapidly, covering a lot of material in a short time. Conversely, the instructor may speak slowly, causing you to become bored and unable to concentrate fully.

Or, the instructor may use jargon or big words without clear meanings, either of which makes understanding the material more difficult and impedes your concentration. Regardless of the reason, you need to learn how to deal with distractions and to concentrate your attention fully on the material under study.

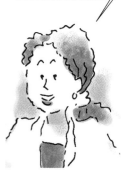

Dealing effectively with distractions can set the foundation for long-term recall of information.

Learning to concentrate

To improve your concentration skills, you must *want* to learn the material. Internal motivation is the key to initiating and maintaining concentration. In addition, you need to be awake and alert, prepared to see, hear, and learn. Being awake and alert allows you to use your class or study time more efficiently and removes the need to review the material a second time when it should have been learned the first time.

Improving your concentration during class and study sessions can help improve retention and foster better scores on tests, quizzes, and assignments.

Eyes front

During class time, try these strategies to help you stay focused:
• Sit up front. The closer you sit to the front, the less distraction between you and the instructor.
• Take a walk between classes to calm down. Walk briskly for 5 to 10 minutes to help ease tension.
• Meditate before class. Find a calm place, close your eyes, sit up straight, relax your arms and legs, and picture something simple, still, and peaceful. Breathe deeply and slowly for about 5 minutes.
• Limit caffeine intake. Caffeine is a central nervous system stimulant. Although a little caffeine can heighten awareness temporarily, too much caffeine can make you jumpy and reduce your ability to concentrate.

Advice from the experts

Meandering mind

Some people seem to remember everything they hear and see, including the entire name of a person they've just met. Others find that their mind tends to wander easily and can't remember as much as they'd like. Do you have a meandering mind? To find out how well you tend to pay attention, ask yourself the questions below. The more you answer yes, the more likely it is that you have a meandering mind and could benefit from strategies to improve your concentration.

• Do you generally forget the names of people you just met?

• Do you find yourself commonly asking people to repeat what they've just said?

• Do you tend to lose track of what's going on, as if you're snapping out of a daydream in the middle of an event?

• Do you sometimes stare blankly at a page?

• Do you sometimes feel as if you don't remember what you've just read, even though you know you read the material?

Study hard

Try these strategies to help improve concentration during study sessions:

• Study when the time is right for you, during periods of alertness.

• Study in a familiar, comfortable place.

• Study under natural light (sunlight) or incandescent light (an ordinary light bulb) rather than fluorescent light to lessen eye strain.

• Set realistic study goals for a study session.

• Make a specific to-do list before you start studying.

• Focus your study on one topic at a time.

• Drink water to prevent dehydration and enhance your ability to maintain focus.

• Vary your study activities. For instance, include in your study time reading, taking notes, and just plain thinking to keep your study process active.

• Take short breaks in your studying every 45 minutes to 1 hour.

• Remove visual distractions from the study area. These distractions can break concentration and stimulate day-dreaming.

• Use an atmosphere of white noise when studying. White noise is a low-level background sound that masks outside distractions. For example, the sound of soft instrumental music can help mask the annoying sound of a clattering air conditioner.

Power napping

If you're having trouble staying awake and alert when studying, try taking a power nap. A short power nap of 5 to 15 minutes — but not longer — can rejuvenate the body and mind. Research indicates that a power nap can replenish the level of amines in the brain. Amines play a role in helping you maintain attention and remain alert and aware.

Improving concentration

There is nothing like practice to improve your concentration. Strategies for improving concentration skills include maintaining a consistent state of mind, reading and relaxing, and thinking globally.

Stress-free learning and recall

If you're relaxed during study, you're more likely to recall information better than if you were tired or stressed when you studied. To reduce stress during studying, keep yourself rested and learn to work within a global framework.

Read and relax

Ideally, you should rest right before a test and before and right after learning new material. Your brain needs time to relax, sort through information, and then store the information for later retrieval. Sleep is particularly important in this regard. During deep sleep, the brain continues to sort and store information, saving important memories and allowing unnecessary ones to be forgotten.

However, keep in mind that during sleep, you can forget important information if your brain hasn't moved it out of short-term memory. Before you go to sleep at night, make a short quiz of 5 to 10 questions from the material you think you've learned. When you wake up in the morning, take the quiz to see how you do. If you've forgotten important information, study it again.

> Rest and relaxation helps your brain learn. Treat rest as a learning tool, not something you don't have time for.

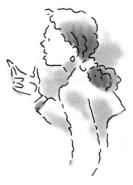

Think globally, study locally

The brain is able to recall information more efficiently when the item being recalled exists within a larger framework of knowledge or more global understanding. For example, a small area of a street map is easier to understand and to recall when considered within the larger framework of a map of the entire city.

In applying this concept to studying, try to learn more about a topic in general before focusing on the particular assigned topic. Television programs, videos, or film documentaries can be good sources of such information. So can magazine articles written for the lay public.

For instance, if you've been assigned a topic of caring for a patient after a coronary artery bypass graft, you might start your studying by reading an article on heart surgery in *Newsweek, Reader's Digest,* or another lay publication. Then, when you read about coronary artery bypass graft in a professional textbook, you'll be able to apply the new knowledge more readily and remember key facts longer.

Memory

Information is stored in different ways and in different forms, which is why you can remember some things clearly and others hardly at all. Memory isn't a sense but a skill that can be developed and improved.

Early memories

Most people can't recall the first year of their life. That's because brain structures responsible for memory don't fully develop until about age 2. In addition, children generally learn to speak after their first year of life, not before. As a result, information stored as memories during the first year of life can't be stored in words.

Some events in childhood, though, remain as clear, vivid memories long after the event has taken place in that person's history. For instance, you clearly remember your first day in school. That's probably because going to school was a new event for you and your brain had to create a new category for it. Later on, going to school became less and less memorable.

I don't remember much about kindergarten, but I remember my first day of elementary school like it was yesterday.

Processing information

How your brain processes memories determines what you remember and what you forget. There are three basic stages involved in information processing:

- registration
- short-term memory
- long-term memory.

Registration

In registration — the initial stage of information processing — information is received and may eventually be understood and selected to be remembered. The process of registration involves three phases: reception, perception, and selection.

What a lovely reception

In reception, you sense something or someone but you don't yet recognize what it is or what it means. For instance, you might auscultate a patient's bowel sounds and hear noises but have no idea what they mean or what condition they represent.

At least, that's my perception

In the second phase, perception, you recognize what you've seen and attach a meaning to it. For example, when auscultating bowel sounds, you hear a whooshing sound. You've already learned in class that a whooshing sound could represent an obstruction of some kind. When you hear the whooshing, you consider that the patient might have an obstruction of some kind. You've attached a meaning to a sound you recognized: that's perception.

Be selective

The final phase of registration involves selection, in which your brain selects information to be remembered. The information selected depends on a number of factors, including the:

- material at hand
- purpose for remembering
- learner's background knowledge
- content and difficulty level of the information
- way the information is organized.

Is it useful?

A person selectively ignores or processes information depending on the usefulness of the information in meeting the person's goals. Information perceived by the learner to be useful tends to be processed. Information perceived to be less useful tends to be ignored.

Ignored information is quickly forgotten; processed information is transferred into short-term memory — the second stage of memory processing.

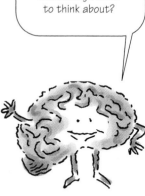

Hmmm, is this something I want to think about?

Short-term memory

All information selected by the brain to be remembered enters short-term memory, which can last as little as 15 seconds. The brain's short-term memory can't hold much information, nor can it hold the information for long. Research indicates that short-term memory can hold five to nine chunks of information, depending on how well the information is grouped.

For example, the numbers 1-8-6-0-1-8-6-4 can be recalled by chunking the numbers into dates — 1860 and 1864. Chunking the information into smaller bits makes it easier to recall the information and allows more memory space for other information.

Chunking up info

When learning new information, your brain has more difficulty organizing, or chunking, the new information because it's unsure of the relationships between pieces of information. That's why learning small chunks of material at a time works better than trying to learn one large chunk all at once.

Wait, there's more

Factors such as age, maturation, amount of practice, meaningfulness of the information, and complexity of information also affect the size of short-term memory. From short-term memory, the brain either forgets the information or moves it to long-term memory.

Long-term memory

After you rehearse and chunk information, your brain can move it to long-term memory. Information stored in long-term memory is organized and stored for long periods, but its duration there depends on how completely the information has been processed and how often you use it. (See *Making memories last.*) Although many techniques can be used to aid in the transfer of information from short-term to long-term memory, the most important one is to use the information right away.

Working memory

Researchers have developed the term *working memory* to describe how your brain stores and retrieves memory from short-term and long-term memory. You can improve your working memory — your ability to store and recall information — through the use of four specific strategies:

- selection
- association
- organization
- rehearsal.

Selection

During selection, choose the information you want to remember and begin selecting ways to process the information. For instance, if you need to learn the steps involved in taking a blood pressure, you need to first decide that the information is important. You know that you'll need to recall the steps in the process in actual practice, so you almost unconsciously decide that the material is important.

Being more consciously aware of what material is important is a key first step in learning the information. When you *really* want to know someone's name, you make a conscious effort to remember it. For instance, you may choose to remember a doctor's last name but not his first name because you'll most likely address him as Dr., not by his first name. Learning new material begins with making a conscious decision to remember it.

Association

After selecting the information you want to remember, create an association to the information. For instance, to remember information about a particular disease, you might associate that material with a patient you once cared for who had the disease. The associations you make

Making memories last

There are many ways to embed what you learn in your long-term memory. Putting the tips listed below into your study regimen can help you retain key information.

Working alone

• Attach a strong emotion to the material.

• Rewrite the material.

• Build a working model of a physical aspect of the material being studied.

• Create a song about the material or change the words to an existing song.

• Draw a picture or create a poster using intense colors.

• Repeat and review the material within 10 minutes, 48 hours, and 7 days.

• Smear a droplet of your favorite perfume onto a reminder note to help you remember the contents of the note.

• Summarize the material in your notes.

• Try to immediately apply what you've learned to activities in your daily life.

• Use mnemonics and acronyms to organize the material.

• Write about the material in a journal.

Working with others

• Act out the material or role-play a situation related to the material being studied.

• Join a study group or other support group.

• Discuss the information with a peer to gain an additional perspective and solidify the material in your mind.

• Make a video or audiotape related to the material being studied.

• Make up and tell a story about the material.

between something you already know and something you're trying to learn serve as memory cues that allow you to more easily retrieve the information later.

Organize

During organization, memorization takes place in an ordered way. You may decide there are too many steps in taking a blood pressure to memorize all at once, so you break the process into smaller chunks, each consisting of only a few steps. Now that the longer list is made up of several smaller steps, you can push the information into long-term memory through repetition. Rewriting the steps, repeating the steps verbally, or role-playing the steps will help you remember the steps more efficiently and clear your working memory for the next piece of new information to be learned. Mnemonics can be particularly effective in organizing chunks of information.

Rehearse

Rehearsal involves repeatedly reviewing information you've learned. Take a tip from the acting profession: One of the best ways to memorize material is to repeat it — or rehearse it — over and over for short periods of time. These short bursts of rehearsal are more effective than long bouts of rehearsal. For example, rather than re-hearsing the steps in taking a blood pressure repeatedly for 1 hour a day, rehearse the steps for 15 minutes 4 times a day. Frequency of rehearsal really pays off when you have a lot of information to remember.

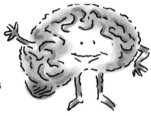

I can push certain memories into long-term storage or just, as they say, fugettuhbout 'em.

Memory retrieval

Once information is processed, it may or may not remain in long-term memory. Information that doesn't remain in long-term memory is forgotten. Information may be for-gotten as a result of infrequent use, depending on how in-terested you are in the information, what your purpose is for learning, how frequently you use the information, and how many connections that memory has made with other pieces of information.

Interested?

In general, the more interested you are in a topic, the stronger the memory of it. For instance, if you know you'll be quizzed on a particular piece of information in anatomy class, you'll be more likely to commit that information to long-term memory. Likewise, purpose, frequency of use, and number of connections all play a role in forming long-term memories.

Now, where did I put that?

The ability to answer questions regarding information you learned a long time ago depends on your ability to recall seldom-used information. (See *Searching for a lost memo-ry.*) Such information may be difficult, or even impossible,

Exercise your mind

Searching for a lost memory

Can't remember something important? Try these strategies to search for a lost memory:

1. Say or write down everything you can remember that relates to the information you're seeking.

2. Try to recall events or information in a different order.

3. Recreate the learning environment or relive the event. Include sounds, smells, details of weather, nearby objects, other people who were present, what you said or thought at the time, or how you felt.

to locate in memory because it hasn't been used in a long time.

To keep your long-term memory ready for challenges, plan a review session once each month. During your review, read aloud your notes from the previous month and add bookmarks to your notes so you can find the content easily later. For instance, if you drew a diagram of the bones of the forearm in your notes, put a note in the margin so you can find the corresponding section of your textbook. If you missed a question on a recent test, highlight and rewrite your notes about the question so you'll know the correct answer the next time. Spending an hour or two each month reviewing information will help keep the information fresh in your mind and keep those synapses firing.

I remember it, but I don't understand it

It's possible for information to be memorized without being understood. With rote memorization, the information can be used only in situations similar to the one in which it was learned. For instance, you might have memorized a concept in chemistry when you were in high school, but because you didn't really understand it, you might find it impossible to apply that learning in your college chemistry class. Understanding a concept, as opposed to just memorizing it, helps to solidify the concept in your long-term memory. You might explain the concept to someone else to bolster your memory even further.

Using the depth gauge

The more deeply a topic is processed by the brain, the more solid is the long-term memory of that topic. Processing depth depends on how the learner processes the information and a number of other factors, including the learner's:

- background knowledge
- desire for learning
- intended use of the information
- intensity of concentration
- level of interest in the topic
- overall attitude.

Study strategies

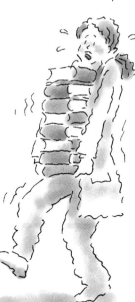

I have all sorts of study strategies at my disposal. It's just that I could use help carrying them.

By using a number of study strategies, you can give yourself the greatest chance to recall information later — on tests or in the clinical area. Using different study strategies gives the brain more pathways to use when recalling information.

Key study strategies include:
- using practice and repetition
- using spaced study
- minimizing interference
- associating familiar items with items to be remembered
- making lists
- using imagery.

Practice

In learning, practice makes permanent. Practice aids the storage of information in long-term memory. It also makes retrieval of information from long-term memory into working memory more automatic.

Rehearsal forms

Practice methods assume many forms, depending on the amount of time spent practicing, the depth of learning that takes place as a result, and the manner in which the information is learned. Rehearsal can take three forms:

Auditory — repeating information aloud or in discussion

Semantic — writing or diagramming information repeatedly

Visual — reading information silently over and over.

Read it aloud

In general, auditory and semantic practices yield better results because they involve active processes rather than the more passive practice of silent reading. Rewriting information while saying it aloud can double your efficiency in learning. Learning takes place more readily as a result of active practices than passive ones.

Spaced study

Spaced study consists of alternating short study sessions with breaks. This method is also known as distributed practice. Study goals are set by time (for example, reading for at least 15 minutes) or task (reading a minimum of three pages). After reaching these goals, the student takes a 5- to 15-minute break.

Why spaced study works

Spaced study works because:
• it rewards hard work
• work is completed in manageable portions
• work is completed under a deadline of time or task, so the time spent studying is spent efficiently
• working memory has limited capacity, so breaks provide time for information to be absorbed into long-term memory
• study breaks keep the student from confusing similar details when studying complex, interrelated information
• separate study sessions are more likely to involve different content cues. The greater the number of study sessions, the greater the likelihood that the content cues overlap with material on the test, thus improving recall.

Interference reduction

Like radio signals creating static, interference occurs when new information conflicts with background knowledge. When two radio signals fall close to one another on the radiowave spectrum, it can be difficult to tune in one fully because of interference with the other. A similar kind of interference occurs in long-term memory. If you have

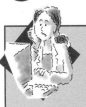

Test-taking tip

Developing associations

Associating information you want to learn with information you already know can help you remember key pieces of information more easily. Use these questions to help you develop associations among study items:

- What, if anything, does the item remind you of?
- Does the item sound like a familiar word or rhyme with one?
- Can you link the item with a memory of a familiar location?
- Can you draw a picture to link your memory with the item?
- When you think of the item, can you visualize something familiar?
- Can you rearrange letters in the name to form an acronym?
- Can you form connections that make sense between one concept and another?

many similar experiences or memories, you may find it difficult to retrieve information about a particular experience or memory.

For instance, if you're trying to learn a large number of new terms and two of the terms are similar, you might have difficulty remembering either. To avoid interference, try to relate new information to previously learned information. Think about what makes the new information different from the previously learned information.

Take a break

If you need to study the subjects one right after the other, at least take a break between the study sessions. When you return to study the second subject, try studying in a different place. Making different associations for each subject will help you and your brain organize information more efficiently.

Associations

To develop the necessary links among information and increase your ability to apply what you've learned, consider how to associate and organize information. (See *Developing associations*.) Applying knowledge to different situations is a critical aspect of learning and requires a deep understanding of the material. Associations form links between familiar items and items to be remembered. When established, the links become automatic.

Recalling a familiar item cues the recall of the other item. To be effective, associations must be personal, perhaps associating a song or smell with the item to be remembered.

Acronyms and acrostics

Forming acronyms or acrostics can prove helpful for recalling lists of information. Acronyms are created from the first letter or the first few letters of each item on a list. *Roy G. Biv* is a commonly used acronym that stands for the colors of the rainbow in order (red, orange, yellow, green, blue, indigo, and violet). *HOMES* is another common acronym, this time for the names of the Great Lakes (Huron, Ontario, Michigan, Erie, and Superior). Acronyms need not be real words.

Acrostics are phrases or sentences represented on the vertical axis and are created from the first letter or first few letters of items on a list. For example, an acrostic representing the lines on the treble clef is *Every Good Boy Does Fine,* which stands for the notes as they appear vertically, from the bottom up, on a treble clef: E-G-B-D-F.

In health care, one of the most famous acrostics is this one (or a variation of it) about the 12 cranial nerves: *On Old Olympus's Towering Tops, A Finn and a Swedish Girl Viewed Some Hops,* which stands for the olfactory, optic, oculomotor, trochlear, trigeminal, abduscens, facial, sensorimotor (vestibulocochlear), glossopharyngeal, vagus, spinal accessory, and hypoglossal nerves.

Acronyms and acrostics each associate key information to an easily remembered word or phrase, thereby improving memory of the information.

Acronyms and acrostics are fun ways of enhancing long-term memory.

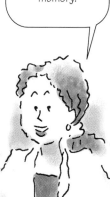

Elaborate, please

Understanding how concepts can be connected with one another helps you learn by allowing for the elaboration of ideas. Elaboration allows you to reframe information in terms of what you already know about the topic. You provide your own logic from your knowledge of how the new information fits with previously learned information.

Lists

Lists serve as another memory aid. The arrangement of a list depends on your goals and the course emphasis and content. Sometimes an instructor suggests organizational structures for lists by identifying types of information to remember — for example, dates, names, and places.

Lists help organize ideas by categorizing information according to some commonality. Recalling the name of the organizing concept helps you remember the details located within it. The organization of information in the list depends on having a classification system of some kind. Because items relate to each other within the system, you can rearrange and reorganize information as needed to aid recall.

Imagery

People commonly think in images rather than words. The use of visual aids in studying can help you recall familiar and unfamiliar information. In addition, images are stored differently in the brain than are words. Imagery provides an additional way to encode information. The brain stores four kinds of memories easily:

- patterns
- pictures
- rhymes
- stories.

Link 'em up

Mental associations link concrete objects with images (for example, a picture of a tree with the word *tree*) or abstract concepts with symbols (for example, a picture of a heart with the word *love*). Mental imagery can also be used to link unrelated objects, concepts, and ideas through visualization. For example, to remember which bone in the forearm is the radius, visualize yourself taking a patient's radial pulse. Then think, the end of the radius is located beneath the radial pulse.

Add a little color

You can use visual representations to help compress and synthesize class notes. Because visual representations of ideas are processed by a different area of the brain than are words, they provide another way to recall information.

Adding meaningful doodles, colors, or symbols to your notes allows you to organize and then visualize information to be learned. A technique called recall mapping can be highly useful in this regard. (See *Recall mapping,* page 52.) When you use visual representations efficiently, you'll remember more information with less effort.

Improving memory skills

You can improve your memory skills through memory-boosting strategies, including:
- writing new information correctly
- using repetition
- using environmental cues
- understanding the information
- developing your own memorization techniques
- using vivid imagery
- having faith in yourself.

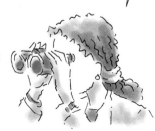

Paying attention to your surroundings can give your memory skills a big boost.

Stay aware

Being aware of everything around you is the first step developing better recall. Be observant. Look for landmarks. Practice being attentive at the big things, and you'll become more attentive at the little ones too.

Register the data

To remember information, the information must first be registered in your brain correctly. If a piece of information

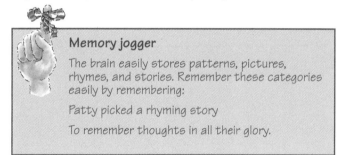

Memory jogger

The brain easily stores patterns, pictures, rhymes, and stories. Remember these categories easily by remembering:

Patty picked a rhyming story

To remember thoughts in all their glory.

Exercise your mind

Recall mapping

Recall mapping is a study technique that uses pictures to enhance memory. For example, you might need to remember a number of health care terms and their definitions. Here's how to perform recall mapping for a series of terms:

• Identify general headings under which the terms might fall.

• List appropriate terms under each heading.

• Draw two lines under each term. On the first line, draw a picture of an object that you can associate with the term or its meaning. On the second line, write the meaning of the term in your own words.

Studying the map

To study the terms using your recall map, cover the information below the term with a sheet of paper, and then try to remember the term's meaning. If you can't remember the meaning, slide the paper away to reveal the picture.

Seeing the drawing should prompt your recall of the meaning. If it doesn't, uncover the definition. Finally, study the term again, recalling why you drew that particular picture. The illustration at right shows an example of a word map.

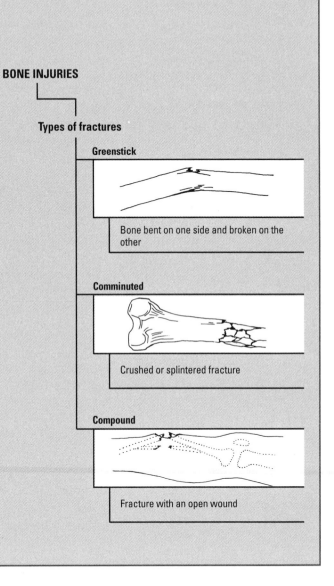

BONE INJURIES

Types of fractures

Greenstick

Bone bent on one side and broken on the other

Comminuted

Crushed or splintered fracture

Compound

Fracture with an open wound

doesn't register, try to expose yourself to the information again. For example, if a new acquaintance's name doesn't register the first time you hear it, ask for the name again. Then repeat it to confirm it.

Understand the information

Make sure you thoroughly understand what you want to remember. Information that makes sense to you and that you fully understand is easier to recall later. To boost your understanding of a topic, use several styles of learning. For instance, don't just read about the radius and ulna. Read about them, watch a video about anatomy, draw a picture of the bones, manipulate your own arm, and talk about the location of the bones with peers. Using various methods of learning can enhance understanding and meaning and, as a result, improve recall.

Let your goals serve as your incentive to study hard and remember more.

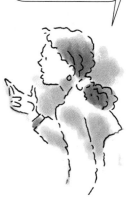

Stay positive and goal-oriented

To intensify your desire to recall information, keep a positive attitude about memory and recall. Believing that you can do something is an important step in actually doing it.

In addition, the more you keep your eyes on your overall goals, the more you can remember. The goal can serve as your incentive to remember information. The stronger the incentive, the stronger the mental connection and longer-lasting the memory.

Use vivid images

To make images in your mind easier to recall, make them more vivid. Think of the colors as being intensely bright. Make the image bigger. Associate a strong emotion to the picture. The more unusual or absurd the mental picture, the more likely that you'll be able to recall the information associated with it.

Here are other ideas for creating vivid images:
• Imagine some kind of action taking place, such as the taking of a pulse.
• Form an image of an object out of proportion to the object's actual size. Make the radius the size of a minivan.
• Exaggerate the object the way a caricature exaggerates the features of its subject.
• Substitute or reverse a normal role. For example, to remember that the radius is located on the thumb side of the forearm, imagine a huge thumb carrying the radius like a dinner tray at a restaurant.
• Practice word associations using mental pictures to remember items in a list. If you need to remember the names of middle ear bones — malleus (also called the hammer), incus (anvil), and stapes (stirrup)— imagine a

cartoonish hammer duking it out with an anvil in a match refereed by a whistle-blowing stirrup. These word associations are memorable because they paint a bizarre picture.

Simple association

Probably the simplest method of remembering a piece of information is by associating the information with something familiar. You can recall one item because another item acts as a reminder. If you wanted to remember to take your anatomy and physiology textbook home to do an assignment, you might place a red self-stick note on your assignment book.

Repetition

Repetition is one of the most effective recall strategies of all. Repetition strengthens neural pathways and, with enough use, can create nearly indelible pathways. Don't depend on repetition alone, however. Use several strategies to make sure the memory remains intact.

Using what works for you

Develop your own favorite memorization techniques, depending on the type of information that needs to be memorized. If you develop a unique memorization technique that works for you, then by all means, continue to use it. As with all techniques, though, remember that you shouldn't rely on a single technique to learn new information, no matter how well that technique has served you in the past. Using a variety of techniques will serve you best in the long run.

Remember that expanding your memorization techniques makes you a more flexible learner, which will allow you to learn a greater variety of material with less stress and wasted time.

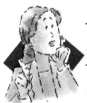

Quick quiz

1. A student's concentration may be impaired by:
   A. being aware of internal distractions.
   B. using mental imagery.
   C. taking scheduled breaks.

Answer: A. Distractions can be external (such as noise) or internal (such as hunger), both leading to impaired concentration.

2. A student who tends to feel pressure and tension during examinations should:
   A. study for her examinations in a tension-free environment.
   B. drink caffeinated beverages before the next examination.
   C. study in the same type of environment that will occur during the next examination.

Answer: C. A student performs better on examinations when she studies under the same conditions that occur during testing. If she tends to feel pressure and tension during an examination, she might benefit from studying under similar conditions.

3. Acronyms are word forms created by combining:
   A. a series of abbreviations in a list into a new word or phrase.
   B. the first letter or first few letters of items on a list into a vertical word or phrase.
   C. the first letter or first few letters of items on a list into a horizontal word or phrase.

Answer: C. Acronyms are created by combining the first letter or first few letters of items on a list into a horizontal word or phrase.

4. The brain stores four kinds of memories easily, including:
   A. dates, pictures, rhymes, and stories.
   B. patterns, numbers, mnemonics, and stories.
   C. patterns, pictures, rhymes, and stories.

Answer: C. Images are stored differently in the brain than are words. The brain tends to store patterns, pictures, rhymes, and stories more easily than other types of information. Using imagery allows your brain to encode information more easily for later recall.

5. To put the process of registration to use when memorizing a person's name, you would:
    A.   ask someone later what the person's name is.
    B.   have the person sign his name.
    C.   repeat the name for verification.
Answer: C. To remember information, the information must be registered in your brain correctly. If a piece of information doesn't register, try to expose yourself to it again, such as by repeating the person's name.

Scoring

☆☆☆   If you answered all five questions correctly, wow! Who can remember a better score?

☆☆   If you answered three or four questions correctly, good show, ol' chap! You deserve entrance into the We'll Never Forget Ya Hall of Fame.

☆   If you answered fewer than three questions correctly, your memory isn't failing; it just needs a little nudge a little nudge a little nudge. (See? We're using repetition here. Yay!)

Part II Successful strategies

4

Time management strategies

Just the facts

In this chapter, you'll learn:

♦ how time management can be used to control and organize your schedule for maximum efficiency

♦ how to set priorities effectively

♦ how to avoid burnout

♦ how procrastination can be overcome by effective planning and a positive approach to projects.

Time assessment

A full-time student spends about 15 hours a week in the classroom and 2 hours of preparation time for each hour of class work — a total of about 45 hours per week involved with school work. Add to that the time required to meet family and financial commitments, and it's easy to see how busy a student's life can be.

Take a student we'll call Shonda, for example. At 37, Shonda has raised three children and has returned to college to finish work toward a degree in nursing. She works 30 hours per week at a bank and attends school every day. A total of 30 hours per week at work, 45 hours per week at school, and dozens of hours per week tending to her home and children make Shonda's life hectic and, at times, disjointed.

With so many responsibilities and so little time to do them, Shonda and every student like her needs to manage time efficiently. To become a more efficient time manager requires an assessment of how time is currently spent.

Exercise your mind

Keeping a time journal

Keeping a journal of how you spend your time can help make you a more efficient time manager. In your journal, keep notes about how alert you feel each day. Keep the time journal for 1 week, and then analyze the data to identify times of good study habits and peak alertness as well as times of bad habits and sluggishness. When creating a schedule, use this analysis to make your downtime work better for you.

Analyze the example

In the example shown below, the student arrives at her anatomy class unprepared, yet she spends time before class talking rather than studying — an inefficient use of her time. What other time management inefficiencies can you spot in this example? What efficiencies can you find? What suggestions would you give this student for improving her time management?

Time	Activity
6:30	Get up. Shower. Dress. Coffee. Tired.
7:00	More coffee. Drive to campus/walk to snack bar. Doughnut. Walk to class. Awake now.
7:55	Talk to classmates in hallway.
8:00	Fundamentals class
9:00	Walk to plaza. Sit in sun. Talk.
9:30	To library. Read 12 pages for anatomy class. Not done. Go to class. Hungry.
10:00	Anatomy class
11:00	Lunch
12:00	Watched game of Frisbee
12:30	Return books to library. Owe library $1.45 in fines. Walk to work.
4:00	Walk home
4:30	Watch rest of Oprah
5:00	Talked to Mike on the phone
6:00	Read 5 pages of Fundamentals. 15 to go
6:30	Read 5 more pages of Anatomy. No time for notes
7:00	Mike here to see movie.
10:00	Home. Too tired to do anything.

Keeping a time journal

To identify areas of inefficient time use, maintain a time journal for 1 week. (See *Keeping a time journal.*) Keep an accurate record of all your activities, described in 30-minute intervals, and include activities throughout the weekend. A time journal will help you identify areas of "dead time," such as that 2-hour stint watching television the other night, and to make the adjustments necessary to manage your time more efficiently.

Schedules

The work habits of people who have achieved outstanding success invariably include a well-designed schedule. When facing several obligations at the same time, it becomes difficult to do any of them. The purpose of scheduling isn't to feel constricted but rather to allow you to look ahead and free yourself from scholastic inefficiency and the anxiety that arises from not being prepared. Developing a course schedule can go a long way toward fulfilling those time management goals.

Getting started

The most successful scheduling technique for most students involves short-range and long-range planning. Develop a general schedule for each marking term, a specific but flexible schedule for each week, and a daily to-do list. The tools you'll need to get started include:
• long-term (semester) calendar that can be posted where you study
• "week-at-a-glance" calendar that includes the current semester
• colorful pens or pencils for color-coding dates and tasks
• notepad or stack of 3″ × 5″ lined cards for daily to-do lists.

Alternatively, you can use an all-in-one organizer system, such as a Day Timer or Day Runner. These systems generally include short-term and long-term calendars and daily to-do lists that can be replaced as needed.

Organizing a class schedule

The way you organize your class schedule affects the success you achieve during the marking term. If you organize your class schedule well, you'll be able to manage your time more effectively. To organize your class schedule properly, spread out class periods throughout the week, schedule difficult classes when you're most alert, strive for a balance between difficult and less-difficult courses each semester, and maintain flexibility throughout the schedule.

Spread the classes around

Some classes are scheduled on alternating days — Monday, Wednesday, and Friday, for instance. Some students may schedule all of their courses on those days, thinking that concentrating their class time and having a day or two free to study makes time management sense. This arrangement, however, often results in being overworked and burned-out on class days and then spending free days recuperating rather than studying. If possible, space your classes throughout the week.

Keep in mind as well that an efficient schedule fills the day as well as the week. Having sufficient time between classes gives you the opportunity to review information as soon as possible after class, which in turn gives you time to think through a lecture while the information is still fresh in your mind.

> Try to balance your schedule between making it too hard and making it too easy.

Tackling the tough classes

Your most difficult courses should be scheduled during the times you're most alert. If you prefer getting up early, schedule your most difficult course for the morning. If you do your best work after lunch, schedule your most difficult classes at that time.

If you have the option of scheduling a class on successive versus alternating days, consider the level of difficulty of the class and how interested you are in it. Difficulty level and interest in a topic affect the length of time you can concentrate on the subject. The more interested you are or the easier the content is for you, the longer you can sustain concentration on the topic.

Magical mix of courses

Although some courses must be taken in sequence, most curricula are somewhat flexible. Generally, course outlines are suggestions about how to spread mandatory and elective courses over 1 or more marking terms. Taking too many difficult courses at once can be overwhelming. Taking too many uninteresting classes can lead to boredom.

To offset either situation, balance courses that you look forward to attending with those you're less interested in, and balance difficult courses with easier courses.

Oh, those commitments

If you're like most students, you have personal commitments (such as holding a full-time or part-time job) or seasonal commitments (such as being a track athlete who trains in the spring). You might also have a hobby that dictates how much time you can devote to course work. Consider these activities and commitments when planning course work, and adjust your course schedule accordingly.

Choose faculty wisely

You might have the option of taking a course with two or more different instructors. If the dates and times of each course fit your schedule, you'll need to decide with which instructor you'd like to take the class. If you don't know the instructors involved, check with other students who might have insight into the teachers or with student government associations, which often monitor faculty performance and make results available to students.

Day-to-day time management

After determining your class schedule for the term, you need to turn your attention to managing your time each day. Start by setting up a calendar to record goals and major events. The purpose of setting up a calendar is to obtain an overview of long-term goals and commitments, which can be helpful in planning short-term and daily activities.

Managing by the year

The calendar should include recreational as well as serious commitments. Using a calendar for the current year, mark off the months and days for the term in which you're currently enrolled. Put the calendar close to where you study so you can focus on your long-term objectives.

Use a calendar to record:

- midterm and final examination dates
- due dates for papers and other projects
- deadlines for completing each phase of lengthy projects
- test dates
- important extracurricular and recreational events
- deadlines for dropping and adding courses
- holidays, school vacations, and social commitments.

> Be especially aware of burnout and procrastination at the beginning and end of a term.

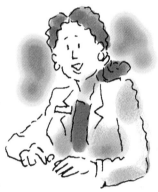

Watch the beginning and the end

The beginning and end of each term are critical times for students. During the first few weeks of a term, the instructor determines the merits of each student. This informal evaluation may become a bias against a student who gets off to a slow start. The end of the term is also critical because the student is running out of time to bring her grades back up if she's fallen behind. Use your calendar to help spot possible distractions during these critical periods. Then plan how to eliminate the distraction or at least reduce its effects.

Avoid study burnout

Burnout results when a student works steadily without taking a sufficient number of breaks. The causes of burnout include fatigue, boredom, and stress. Maintaining a balance between breaks and work time helps avoid burnout.

To avoid burnout, plan for breaks as well as study time. A break doesn't have to be recreational; it can be a change from one task to another. For example, switching from an anatomy assignment to a reading assignment in your fundamentals textbook can relieve boredom and, thus, prevent burnout. Such planning also decreases interruptions during prime study time.

Another way to avoid burnout is to retain flexibility in your daily schedule. If you schedule commitments too tightly during the day, you won't have time to complete

Exercise your mind

Developing a weekly calendar

Every Sunday, make it a habit to complete the coming week's calendar with academic and social commitments. Below is a 3-day sample of a typical student's weekly calendar. What advice would you give this student to make more efficient use of her time?

Monday		Tuesday		Wednesday	
8:00 to 9:00	Fundamentals class	7:30 to 9:00	Study for dosage calc test. Do sample problems.	8:00 to 9:00	Fundamentals class
9:00 to 9:30	Review notes.			9:00 to 9:30	Review Fund. notes.
9:30 to 11:00	Read 20 pages in Med-Surg for Friday.	9:00 to 10:30	Dosage calc test	9:30 to 11:00	Read 20 pages in Med-Surg.
		10:30 to noon	Read 20 pages in Med-Surg. Start research for lab assignment.	11:00 to Noon	A & P class
11:00 to Noon	Med-Surg class			8:00 to 9:30	Finish research for lab assignment.
2:00 to 5:00	Baseball game	1:00 to 2:00	Lab		
7:30 to 9:30	Study for dosage calc test. Do sample problems.	3:00 to 7:00	Work		
		8:30 to 10:00	Laundry. Review Med-Surg.		

your goals and, as a result, may feel defeated for failing to do what you had planned.

Managing by the week

Maintaining a weekly calendar helps you keep on track not just for the week but for the entire marking term as well. (See *Developing a weekly calendar.*) When constructing a weekly calendar, keep these guidelines in mind:

• List fixed commitments — such as weekly or unbreakable appointments — first.

• Set aside a few minutes before each class to review notes and preview that day's topic.

• Take a few minutes after each class to review the notes you just took and material you just covered.

• Look for and implement more efficient ways to group activities together. Grouping similar activities together can save time and improve overall efficiency.

• Plan to complete activities before the final due date to allow for unexpected delays.

• Schedule study periods for 50 to 90 minutes at a time, interspersed with a 15-minute break.
• Schedule a sufficient amount of time for studying. Be realistic. Figure that you'll spend 2 hours of out-of-class study for every hour of in-class time.
• Study at the same time every day.
• Make effective use of open time during the school day, particularly between classes. When you find yourself with free time, pull out a textbook or your notes and complete studying you might otherwise have delayed until later.
• Set aside at least 1 hour each week (not regularly scheduled study time) for a review of each class period and what you need to prepare for the class.
• Leave some time unscheduled for added flexibility.

What's this week's game plan?

When constructing a weekly calendar, first block out fixed commitments, including class time, mealtimes, and sleep time, among others. Allow a reasonable amount of time for each activity. For example, daily travel times differ according to the time of day, amount of traffic, and route taken. You might schedule 30 minutes to travel one way to school and 45 minutes to travel the other way.

Be specific about how you use your time. Complete your schedule at the beginning of each week, preferably on Sunday, when you can look ahead to the coming week. Your weekly schedule should include homework assignments, papers due, and upcoming tests. Homework that hasn't been assigned yet can be anticipated. For instance, if you know you're supposed to read a chapter each week in pharmacology class, note this goal on your schedule.

Every Sunday, I use an electronic planner to plan the coming week. Then I print it out as a reference.

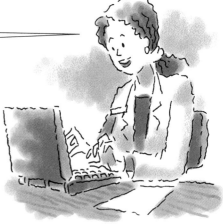

Exercise your mind

Making a to-do list

Your daily to-do list itemizes the personal and academic things you want to accomplish that day. The list below shows typical entries on a to-do list. What entries would your to-do list have on it today?

To do today
Study for dosage calc test
Dosage calc test
Read 20 pages in A & P
Review catheterization for lab practical
Start research for lab assignment
Work at hospital
Laundry

By coordinating activities and assignments and spreading them out during the week, you can avoid having too much to do on a single day. In addition, you can look ahead to avoid conflicts, rescheduling activities when necessary.

Managing by the day

After completing your weekly calendar, construct the next day's to-do list by organizing your goals for the day. Working from the weekly calendar, list all the items you want to complete the next day. Don't include standard tasks, such as eating, sleeping, or attending class.

Do, however, include such tasks and assignments as "Read 20 pages of *History of Nursing: Part II*." Check the task off when you've accomplished it or, if you read only 10 pages rather than 20, add the remaining pages to the next day's or week's reading. (See *Making a to-do list*.)

To manage time effectively, stay flexible.

Building in flexibility

Keep in mind when setting up a daily schedule that you don't have to plan every minute of every hour of every day, nor do you have to be militant about sticking to your schedule. To maintain maximum time efficiency, be flexible. Routines are important, but so is flexibility.

Earning rewards

Small rewards given for small achievements serve as an incentive for sticking to a schedule. Crossing off an item on your daily to-do list can give you a sense of satisfaction in completing a task. Make it a point to give yourself a small reward for each small task completed during the day. Give yourself a larger reward for finishing a larger project, making sure the reward is appropriate to the task.

Perhaps you can reward yourself with 5 minutes of free time. Or, put a set amount of money into a jar every time you finish one part of a large project. Give yourself all the money in the jar when you finish the entire project.

Set up the rewards in advance. Deny yourself something you want until after you've accomplished a task. For example, don't allow yourself to call friends until after you've read the chapter you scheduled yourself to read.

Setting priorities

Setting priorities is a critical task for every student. You'll need to set priorities appropriately in school and in the clinical area as well. You'll need to set priorities for tasks, class attendance, and homework.

Tasks

A student with several tasks that have the same deadline may switch back and forth from one task to another, giving the illusion of progress. Changing tasks too often, however, wastes time because you lose momentum. For a time after the transition from one project to another, you may still be thinking about the old project when you should be concentrating on the new one. Furthermore, after returning to the first task, you have to review where you were and what steps remained before the task could be finished.

So little time, so many tasks

You can avoid this problem by determining how much time you have available in any one period. If you have an hour or less available, work on only one task. Only if you have more than an hour should you alternate tasks. Even then, most of your attention should be focused on completing a single task (or a large portion of it), which can provide a sense of satisfaction and move you steadily toward completion of your goals.

If you interrupt work on a long-term project to work on another task, write a few notes about the long-term project before moving to the new task. Write down the goal of the task and a list of questions to be answered or objectives to be completed. You might jot down what steps you plan to perform next so that, when you return to the task, you can pick up where you left off right away. Be sure as well to store all materials related to the first task in the same place so you don't have to search for materials when you return to the task.

Attending class

During class, the instructor highlights the most important concepts, elaborates on information found in assigned readings, and shapes the student's understanding of the material. Instructors focus on application, analysis, and synthesis of ideas in their lectures and classroom work. The instructor uses class time to present the material she thinks is most important for understanding the course.

To get the most out of class time, arrive on time and don't leave early. Instructors often use the first 5 minutes of class to make important announcements and the last 5 minutes to summarize material or explain an assignment. Bring other

> I usually cover important information at the beginning of class. If you miss it, you put yourself at a disadvantage.

assignments or readings to class in case the teacher is late or you have an unexpected break.

Be there or be, um, just *be there*

Missing a class is risky. Each time you miss a class, you face the possibility that questions on the next test will relate to material covered in the class you missed. In addition, many students assume they can safely miss a class here and there because they pay close attention to their reading assignment.

The problem with that approach is that many instructors don't use only the reading material to construct lecture notes and create classroom activities and discussions. They commonly base classroom material on their own experiences and on sources not readily available to the student, such as journal articles, educational newsletters, and other nontextbook sources of information.

Even if an instructor bases her classroom activities entirely on textbook readings, you would still miss explanations of new ideas and the further development of existing content. Here's another reason not to skip class: Learning continues outside the classroom. After class, you continue to think about the material. You might be walking home from class, showering, or doing the laundry when you come up with a question to ask or clarify in your mind a statement made in class. Just because your body is no longer located in a classroom doesn't mean your brain has finished analyzing material covered in that classroom. Give your mind a chance to help you learn; attend every class.

> Try never to miss a class. But if it can't be helped, try to borrow a classmate's notes.

The bitter end

The worst time to miss a class is at the end of the semester. Some instructors use the last few classes of the semester to review and outline the entire course or to discuss information to be covered on the final examination. Some instructors even go so far as to tell — or at least hint at — exactly what material the students should study for the final examination.

Even so, some students feel overwhelmed with studying for final examinations and end up trading class time for study time. If you schedule your study time well, you can avoid feeling the need to skip class to study. If you're truly unable to attend a class, however, ask another student if you can borrow her notes and get copies of classroom handouts for that day. That way, you'll at least be exposed to some of the material covered in class.

Doing homework

Homework assignments typically fall into two categories: written or reading assignments. Written assignments provide an instructor with immediate feedback about how much work the student has done and how well she has understood it.

Although reading assignments don't provide immediate feedback, instructors generally consider them equally as important for understanding a particular subject. Many instructors include questions on reading assignments on quizzes and tests or ask questions in class based on assigned readings. The responses of the students help the instructor gauge the effectiveness of the assignment and whether the students have actually read the material.

Eh, what's next, Doc?

To gain the most value from homework assignments, you first need to find out what the assignments are for the course. Most instructors distribute a syllabus or an outline at the start of each course. These documents explain content to be covered in the course and what expectations the instructor has for the student. Some instructors also distribute reading and written homework assignments for each course. If you don't receive such an outline, approach your instructor and ask what material you should read for the next few classes. Then create your own outline, and put the assignments into your organizer so you can plan your daily and weekly schedule properly.

Don't put low-priority tasks ahead of high-priority ones.

Postponing homework

Family and other responsibilities sometimes take precedence over school work. In those situations, try to balance your schedule by not overdoing it in one area at the expense of another. Postponing certain homework assignments for a short time might free up enough time to fulfill family obligations or other responsibilities. Having the support of your employer, fellow workers, and family can prove critical in this regard. However, avoid postponing homework routinely. Doing so can put you so far behind in your studies that you won't be able to catch up.

Advice from the experts

Breaking the procrastination habit

Procrastination habits can be hard to break but not impossible. To break your procrastination habits, follow the tips below.

Motivators

• On one side of a sheet of paper, write your reasons for not doing something On the other side, challenge the excuse with logic. For example, if your reason for not starting your Dosage Calculations project is that you're not in the mood, you might counter with, "Well, you may *never* be in the mood and the job will *never* get done unless you do it."

• Make up a list of self-motivating statements, such as "It's now or never," "No time like the present," or "Never put off until tomorrow what you should do today." Then repeat them whenever you feel like postponing a task.

• Recognize that the negative predictions you might make about a project aren't facts. Focus on the positive steps you can take toward reaching your goals, no matter how difficult those goals might be.

• Commit to complete each task. Promise yourself, a friend, or a relative that you'll get the task done. A promise to a third person can serve as a powerful motivator.

Goals and priorities

• Design clear goals, and then establish a realistic timetable to complete each one.

• Set priorities. Write down all the things that need to be done for a project in order of their importance. The greater the importance, the higher the priority.

• Break down large, complex projects into smaller, more manageable parts. For example, make an outline for a written report before composing it.

• Use your weekly schedule and daily to-do lists to keep yourself organized. Check off tasks after completion.

• Pinpoint where your delays typically start, and then focus on overcoming procrastination during those critical times.

• Write reminders to yourself about projects to be completed, and display them in conspicuous places.

Rewards

• Reward yourself. Self-reinforcement can have a powerful effect on developing a "do it now" attitude.

• Promise yourself to give up something important if you fail to meet your goal and to go someplace special if you *do* meet your goal.

Handling procrastination

Everyone procrastinates, some more so than others. In the end, procrastination results in wasted time, missed opportunities, poor performance, self-deprecation, and increased stress. Procrastinators often spend more time worrying than working.

People who procrastinate place low-priority tasks ahead of high-priority ones and then offer excuses for not doing the high-priority task, including:
- I'll wait until I'm in the mood.
- I feel like celebrating because I finished reading one chapter.
- I'll think about it tomorrow.
- There is plenty of time to get it done.
- I don't know where to begin.
- I work best under pressure.
- I've got too many other things to do first.

Students may procrastinate to avoid tasks that seem boring or difficult, or they may put off working on a task because they doubt their ability to do the task to begin with. In addition, a student may wait until all available resources have been reviewed before completing a task. Regardless of the cause, procrastination needs to be identified and then overcome to succeed as a student. (See *Breaking the procrastination habit.*)

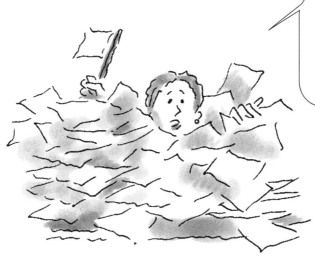

I've broken up 18 large tasks into about a gazillion smaller parts so I can focus on finishing one part at a time. Gee, do I feel better. Uh-huh.

Give it a try

When you recognize that you're procrastinating, try doing for just a few minutes what you're thinking about postponing. Once you've started the task, you're likely to continue working on it.

Parcel it out

When you face several deadlines in the same week, it can be difficult to prioritize and get started on a task. In these cases, parcel the work, setting apart small tasks that can be accomplished quickly. Completing several small tasks provides positive reinforcement and moves you closer and closer to your goal.

Set realistic goals

Some students fail to start projects because the students set impossibly high standards and are afraid they won't live up to their own expectations. Other students refuse to finish a project until they believe it's perfect, a goal they may never reach. In either case, you should weigh the consequences of handing in what you believe is a flawed project with the consequences of not handing in a project at all. Understand that a passing grade for an imperfect assignment beats a zero for not handing in an assignment at all. Use this knowledge as an impetus for getting the project completed at all costs.

Concentration without distractions

The student who can't concentrate enough to get started on a project, and so puts off starting on the project, needs to remove the distractions from her study area or move to an area where there are fewer distractions. When undertaking a project, make sure that reference materials are nearby so that you don't interrupt your work flow to find a particular resource.

Be decisive

Sometimes uncertainty can cause apathy and indecisiveness and, consequently, procrastination. For instance, if you're not sure which topic you should choose for a project, you'll have a harder time making a commitment to the project and an easier time putting off getting started. To avoid procrastination due to uncertainty, keep in mind that decisiveness is a trait of an effective leader and a successful student. Brainstorming for ideas with other students, asking your instructor for suggestions on a topic, or researching several topics that might interest you can help you decide on a topic and move you toward fulfilling your goals.

Review your goals

Lack of clear, specific goals is often a subtle cause of procrastination. If you're unsure of your goals, you'll have little reason to begin or complete a project. Likewise, if you become so involved in working on one assignment, you may forget due dates for other commitments. Establishing long-term and short-term goals — and then periodically reviewing them — can help provide direction to the tasks you perform and keep you on track during unusually busy periods.

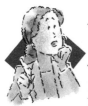

Quick quiz

1. A student who prefers arising early should schedule her most difficult course:

    A. in the morning.

    B. right after lunch.

    C. in the afternoon or early evening.

Answer: A. If a student prefers getting up early, she should schedule her most difficult course for the morning, when she's most alert.

2. Each study period you schedule should last:

    A. 15 to 30 minutes.

    B. 30 to 45 minutes.

    C. 50 to 90 minutes.

Answer: C. Schedule study periods for 50 to 90 minutes at a time with a 15-minute break.

3. The worst time to miss a class is the:

    A. beginning of a semester.

    B. end of a semester.

    C. middle of a semester.

Answer: B. The worst time to miss a class is at the end of the semester. Some instructors use the last few classes of the semester to review and outline the entire course or to discuss information to be covered on the final examination.

Scoring

☆☆☆   If you answered all 3 questions correctly, you're stupendous! You've climbed to the peak of Mt. Efficiency!

☆☆   If you answered 2 questions correctly, good for you. You've scaled Scheduler's Summit.

☆   If you answered fewer than 2 questions correctly, that's OK. We have faith that you'll be climbing Nonprocrastinator's Peak in no time!

Stress management strategies

Just the facts

In this chapter, you'll learn:

♦ that stress is the body's response to a demand

♦ how the body responds to stress

♦ why anxiety is the most common study-related stress symptom

♦ how stress management techniques can be directed at the body or the mind.

What is stress?

Stress, according to the famed neuropsychologist Hans Selye, is "the nonspecific response of the body to any demands made upon it." When faced with a stimulus, the body seeks to adapt. These adaptations provoke a variety of physical and psychological reactions that, collectively, we recognize as stress.

People typically think of stress as being negative or unpleasant, but that's not the case. We can react to stress positively or negatively, depending on the type of stress and our ability to manage it.

Eureka! Eustress!

People commonly encounter situations that cause them to react in a positive way. This response to beneficial environmental stimuli, called eustress, helps keep us alert, motivates us to face challenges, and drives us to solve problems. These low levels of stress are manageable and can be thought of as necessary and normal stimulation.

Distress = damage

Distress, on the other hand, results when our bodies over-react to events. Distress leads to what has been called the fight-or-flight response, a reaction deeply rooted in human physiology and behavior. The fight-or-flight response evolved as a mechanism to deal with life-or-death situations faced by primitive humans.

Nowadays, truly life-or-death situations tend to occur rarely for most people. Yet, the human body continues to react to day-to-day situations the way our ancestors did, as if our lives depended on our reactions. For instance, your body can't physiologically differentiate between the threat of a saber-toothed tiger and that of a boss in a gray tweed suit. How we perceive and interpret the events of life dictates how our body reacts. If we think something is scary or worrisome, our bodies react accordingly.

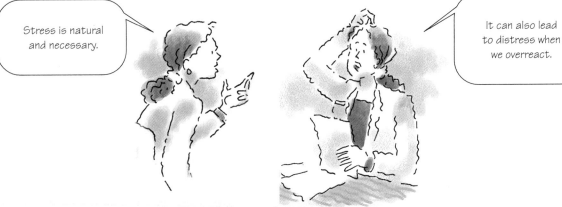

Stress is natural and necessary.

It can also lead to distress when we overreact.

Rating your reaction

Exposing two people to the same stressor can provoke very different reactions. One possible explanation for these differences is that people have varying levels of what psychologists call coherence, or a sense of fitting into the environment. People with a strong sense of coherence feel more in control of themselves and react more positively to stress than do people with a weaker sense of coherence. Understanding how you tend to react to stress can help you gain control of your reactions and cope with stress more effectively.

Reacting to stress

Selye categorized the body's reactions to environmental stress in three phases, together called the general adaptation syndrome (GAS). The phases of GAS are:

- alarm
- resistance
- exhaustion.

> Stress alerts my hypothalamus, which activates the autonomic nervous system and sets body defenses in motion.

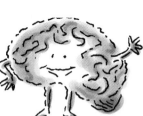

Reaction

In the first stage, alarm, a nonspecific, general alarm occurs. In this response, the hypothalamus in the brain activates the autonomic nervous system, which in turn sparks activity in the pituitary gland and leads to an arousal of body defenses. At this point, the person experiences an increase in alertness and anxiety.

Resistance

During the second phase of the GAS, resistance, the hormone epinephrine is released from the adrenal glands. Epinephrine helps the body counteract the stressor directly or take flight to avoid the stressor's harmful effects.

Exhaustion

If exposure to the same stressor continues over a long period, the body will no longer be able to adapt to or resist the stressor's effects, and exhaustion sets in. Regardless of the inner strength of an individual, prolonged, unrelenting stress eventually breaks down the body's resistance, and disease, or even death, can result.

What stress looks like

Signs and symptoms of stress vary, depending on whether the stress reaction is of short duration or prolonged. Stress can also cause a number of psychological effects.

Short-term stress

Short-term signs and symptoms of stress are easy to recognize and differ little from person to person. When faced with stress, the person's:
- breathing becomes rapid and shallow

• heart rate increases
• muscles in the shoulders, forehead, and back of the neck tighten
• hands and feet become cold and sweaty.

Stress can also lead to disturbances in the GI system, such as a "butterfly" stomach or diarrhea, vomiting, and frequent urination. The mouth may become parched, and the hands and knees may begin to shake or tremble. These short-term effects disappear soon after the stressor is removed.

Prolonged stress

Extended exposure to stress can have lasting or even permanent effects on the body. Chronic stress suppresses the immune system by destroying white blood cells (WBCs) and suppressing WBC production, thus diminishing the body's disease-fighting capabilities. In addition, stress causes the release of free fatty acids into the bloodstream. These fatty acids can eventually accumulate as fatty deposits on arterial walls and lead to coronary artery disease, stroke, or heart attack.

Matters of the mind

A number of psychological changes also occur due to stress. Memory becomes blocked, and clear thinking becomes difficult. A stressed individual may also find it difficult to solve problems efficiently. If the situation persists, the person finds it difficult to concentrate and may experience a general sense of fear or anxiety, insomnia, early waking, changes in eating habits, excessive worrying, fatigue, or a frequent urge to escape from the stressor.

A small amount of stress helps me focus.

Characteristics of anxious students

Stress from classroom and test situations commonly results in anxiety. (See *Coping with test-taking anxiety.*) Study-related anxiety can affect your performance as a student in several ways. Anxiety appears to improve performance on simple tasks and heavily practiced skills but it interferes with the accomplishment of more complex tasks or skills that aren't thoroughly practiced.

If simple, practiced skills have become boring or rote, a small amount of

Advice from the experts

Coping with test-taking anxiety

A test may cause undue anxiety. If you're experiencing worry and anxiety before a test, you can use a number of techniques to help you cope more effectively with test-taking anxiety.

Before the test

• Discuss test content with your instructor and classmates.

• Develop effective study and test preparation skills.

• Spread your final studying over several days rather than cramming right before the test.

• Review your textbook, notes, and homework problems.

• Jot specific concepts or formulas on 3″ × 5″ cards and then study the cards.

• Take a practice test under examlike conditions.

• Continue your regular exercise program.

• Get sufficient rest the night before the test.

• Emphasize positive aspects of the test when you find yourself thinking negatively.

• Avoid studying immediately before the test.

• Relax or do something non-test-related immediately before the test.

• Arrive at the testing room about 5 minutes early to relax before the test is distributed. Arriving earlier than that may cause undue anxiety.

During the test

• Do something to break the test atmosphere, if allowed, such as getting a drink, sharpening a pencil, eating a snack, or asking a question.

• Alternately tense and relax muscles in several parts of your body, and then take several deep breaths with your eyes closed.

• Practice calming yourself by saying something like, "I have much more in my life than this test. I am calm and relaxed."

• Visualize a calm, soothing scene whenever you feel anxious.

anxiety can help keep you alert and eager to finish. If a task is difficult or new, however, anxiety can prove distracting, making it more difficult to complete the task successfully.

Advice from the experts

Recognizing the "freeze-up"

The most common symptom of test anxiety is experiencing a mental block or "freeze-up." A person with test anxiety may read the test questions and find the words meaningless. Or, the person may need to read test questions several times to fully comprehend them. Other symptoms include:

• feeling panic about not knowing the answer to a question or as time is running out of the test period

• worrying how your performance compares to the performance of other students

• feeling easily distracted during the examination

• plotting ways to escape from a test, such as sneaking out or faking an illness.

Misplaced attention

Highly anxious students seem to divide their attention between the new material and a preoccupation with how nervous they're feeling. So instead of concentrating on a lecture or on what they're reading, anxious students keep noticing the tight feelings in their chest, thinking something like, "I'm so tense, I'll never understand this stuff!" Because much of an anxious student's attention is occupied with negative thoughts about performing poorly, being criticized, or feeling embarrassed, she may miss much of the information she's supposed to learn.

Avoid the "freeze and forget." Learn stress management skills.

Occupied by irrelevant details

Anxious students tend to have poor study habits. They commonly have trouble learning material if it's somewhat disorganized or difficult to understand or if it requires them to rely on their memory. Anxious students may be more easily distracted by irrelevant or incidental aspects of the task at hand. They seem to have trouble focusing on significant details and, as a result, waste a great deal of time.

Freeze and forget

Anxious students often know more than they can demonstrate on a test, but because they commonly lack effective test-taking skills, they fail to demonstrate their knowledge.

They "freeze and forget" in a testing environment even though they might excel in nontest environments. (See *Recognizing the "freeze-up."*)

Managing stress

Stress management is an activity that can occur on many levels. It can be as simple as taking a 5-minute break from studying and as comprehensive as reconsidering your life goals. To truly adjust your reaction to stress, choose the kinds of stress management techniques that will work for you. These techniques include:
- setting priorities
- caring for the body
- caring for the mind
- using social supports.

Setting priorities

A key factor in stress management involves managing the limited amount of time you have. As a student, the chores you need to fit into each day may include going to classes, studying and preparing for class, working, participating in extramural activities, fulfilling family responsibilities, engaging in your favorite hobbies, exercising, or attending social affairs.

Feeling the burden of fitting all those activities into a limited time is a source of significant stress. Setting priorities can help you manage activities and reduce the stress they cause.

Simplify your life

It seems that we're always faced with more to do than can be accomplished. At times you may feel overwhelmed with responsibility, overextended, and out of control. The answer to a life that seems overwhelming is simplification. As Elaine St. James, a leader of the simplicity movement, states in her book, *Simplify Your Life,* "Wise men and women in every major culture throughout history have found that the secret to happiness isn't in getting more but in wanting less." She encourages everyone to take some time out, examine their life, and set some reasonable and specific goals that will simplify life.

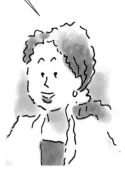

Set priorities to help you manage day-to-day activities and reduce stress.

Simplifying your life means identifying what you most want to have and most want to accomplish. Then determine how to reach those goals as simply as possible. For example, you may want to buy an expensive new car. Do you also want the high insurance rates that come with it? Are you ready for the added drain on your family's finances? Or would you prefer at this point to buy a solid, dependable secondhand car?

Other ways to simplify your life include:

• Run your errands all in one place. Don't hop from one shopping center to another. That takes time and energy. You might have to pay a little more for some of the things you need, but it will be worth it by making one stop instead of five or six.

• Turn off the television.

• Don't answer the phone every time it rings. If you have an answering machine, let it pick up sometimes. Give yourself a break.

• Stop sending greeting cards at Christmas and other holidays.

• Resign from organizations whose meetings you hate to attend.

• Say no to one request each day or week.

• Every once in a while, just do nothing.

Remember, life isn't a race. Take it at your own pace, and simplify.

Spread out the schedule

If you can't reduce the number of demands you have, try to increase the time you allow yourself to perform them. Many deadlines are self-imposed. If you're overscheduled in your classes and, as a result, overwhelmed with responsibilities, perhaps you can aim to graduate a semester later. Sometimes it's necessary to differentiate between deadlines that can't be changed and those that can be extended without compromising goals.

Undo the urgency

It's easy to mistake an urgency for an emergency. When you're feeling overwhelmed, sit down and divide a sheet of paper into three columns. Label the columns *Emergency, Urgency,* and *Non-urgent.* Then prioritize all the tasks on your to-do list according to whether they're true emergencies (things that *must* be done immediately), urgencies (things that are important but aren't emergencies), or non-urgent. A bathtub that's leaking water through the ceiling into the kitchen is an emergency; handle it right away. If the tub is partly plugged but still drains and isn't leaking, it's urgent; handle it as soon as you have time. A bathtub that works fine but needs to be cleaned is non-urgent; handle it the next time you clean the bathroom.

Tasks that don't fit into any of the columns aren't important. Take them off your list, or put them on a separate list titled, "Things to do sometime, maybe." Above all, keep other people's needs in mind but don't sacrifice your needs and your health for things that aren't emergencies or urgencies.

> I've got a long essay to write, but for now I'm focusing on completing the introduction. That's my priority today.

Arranging the sock drawer isn't a high priority

Organize your schedule to make the most of what time is available. Identify and reduce wasted time, delegating certain activities to others in your social network and avoiding taking on too much yourself. Eliminate tasks if they aren't a high priority. That way you can schedule more time for high-priority tasks.

Allow for imperfections

Another problem that affects optimal use of time is striving for perfection with each task, thereby delaying the task's completion. Give yourself permission to be imperfect. Not every task requires perfect effort. That doesn't mean you should do sloppy work, but it does mean that you should avoid laboring over tasks until the outcome is what you consider perfect.

Start small

Be aware of procrastination that stems from feeling unable to complete a task. If a task seems overwhelming, break it down into smaller tasks that can be done individually. It's better to start with a small step than not to start at all.

Caring for the body

Because stress prompts a physical response from the body, caring for the body properly plays an important role in your ability to effectively manage stress. Caring for the body involves exercising, getting proper rest, eating well, and using stress-reducing breathing activities.

Exercise

Many students complain about not having enough time to study, let alone to exercise. However, finding the time to exercise — even if it's just a daily regimen of stretches in the morning — can help lower stress, keep you looking and feeling trim, and make you feel better all around. Rather than draining energy, regular exercise actually replenishes your energy supply, allowing you to more easily manage all of the tasks you need to complete each day. Knowing what kinds of activities are best and how long and how often to exercise are the first steps on the path to a healthy body.

Swim, jog, walk, or bike

Aerobic activities, such as swimming, jogging, brisk walking, cycling, or engaging in a vigorous racquet sport, not only strengthen your cardiovascular system, but also provide numerous other physiologic benefits. For instance, people who engage in aerobic exercise tend to have more energy, feel less stress, sleep better, lose weight more easily, and experience an improved self-image.

In choosing the type of exercise you do, select an activity you enjoy. Unless you enjoy it, you won't continue with it. You might also look for an exercise partner to provide companionship, camaraderie, and motivation to exercise on a regular basis.

Three times a week, 20 minutes per time

Exercise at least three times a week for at least 20 to 30 minutes at a time. You'll see even greater improvements if you build gradually to four to six times weekly. Give yourself at least one day per week free of exercise so your body can rest properly.

Rest

People experiencing high levels of stress tend to get insufficient amounts of sleep and become fatigued. Fatigue by itself is a stressor, which increases the amount of stress you feel, which leads to more fatigue, and so on. Sometimes it's more important to get some rest than to complete every task on your daily to-do list. Listen to your body when it tells you it's tired. Like that

Getting sufficient rest is an important stress management tool.

famous brokerage firm commercial, when your body talks, you should listen.

Eating right

A balanced, nutritious diet is essential for maintaining good health. Diet also may influence your ability to cope with stress. Studies have shown that eating an adequate breakfast each day can improve the body's reaction to stress. Hunger can make an individual less able to cope effectively with stress.

Go for fruits and vegetables

During periods of stress, increase your intake of fruits and vegetables to supply vitamins B and C and folic acid, all of which enhance your body's ability to deal with the stress. Foods that can help elevate your mood include those that contain the amino acid tryptophan, such as milk, eggs, poultry, legumes, nuts, and cereal.

Go decaf and de-sugar

Reducing your consumption of coffee, tea, cola soft drinks, or drugs containing caffeine can help control stress. Caffeine stimulates the sympathetic nervous system and promotes tension and anxiety. Avoid high-glucose foods as well; they can lead to sudden increases and decreases in blood glucose, which affect your ability to concentrate.

Herbs for energy

Ginseng, a popular herb, and another herb called mugwort are thought to improve stress resistance when taken for short periods. However, no studies have proven the effectiveness of either herb for this use. In addition, mugwort can cause anaphylaxis.

Stress-reduction techniques

A number of stress-reduction techniques can be used to counteract your body's damaging reactions to stress, including conscious relaxation, massage, relaxation breathing, and yoga and other meditation-based activities.

Unwind those muscles

Relaxation is a conscious attempt to relax your muscles. Because tension tends to target muscles in the head, neck, and shoulders, many relaxation techniques focus on those parts of the body.

Here's an example of one relaxation technique. Relax your neck and shoulders. Slowly drop your head forward, roll it gently to the center of your right shoulder, and pause. Gently roll it to the center of your left shoulder, and pause. Roll it gently forward to the center of your chest, and pause. Reverse direction and go from left to right. Your goal for this and other forms of conscious relaxation is to slowly stretch muscles into relaxation. Similar techniques can be used to relax your entire body. (See *Full-body relaxation*.)

Therapeutic massage

Therapeutic massage today is used primarily for stress reduction and relaxation. The primary physiologic effect of therapeutic massage is improved blood circulation and muscle relaxation. As the muscles are kneaded and stretched, blood return to the heart increases and toxins such as lactic acid are carried out of the muscle tissue to be excreted from the body.

Improved circulation also results in increased perfusion and oxygenation of tissues. Improved oxygenation of the brain helps us think more clearly and, psychologically, to feel relaxed and more alive. Massage also appears to trigger the release of endorphins, the body's natural pain relievers.

Qigong

Qigong (pronounced "chee goong") is a system of gentle exercise, meditation, and controlled breathing used by millions of Chinese people daily to increase strength and relax the mind. Practitioners believe that when practiced daily over time, *qigong* can improve strength and flexibility, reverse damage due to injury or disease, relieve pain, restore energy, and induce relaxation and healing.

There's nothing like a massage to relax stressed-out muscles. Aaaaaah.

Advice from the experts

Full-body relaxation

Relaxation exercises not only reduce stress, but also send more blood and oxygen to the muscles. As muscles relax, they stretch, which allows more blood to flow into them. As a result, they gradually feel warmer and heavier. To relax your entire body in an attempt to reduce stress, try this exercise.

Start at the feet
Begin by settling back into a comfortable position. Start by focusing on relaxing your feet and ankles. Wiggle your feet or toes to help them to relax, and then allow that wave of relaxation to continue into the muscles of the calves. Continue the process up to the muscles of the thighs. Your legs should gradually feel more and more comfortable and relaxed.

Upper body
Next, concentrate on relaxing the muscles of your spine. Feel the relaxation spread into your abdomen. As you do this, you might feel a pleasant sense of warmth spreading to other parts of your body.
 Focus on the muscles of the chest. Each time you exhale, your chest muscles should relax a little more. Let this relaxation flow into the muscles of the shoulders and then the arms and hands. Gradually, your arms and hands will become heavy, limp, and warm.

Neck and head
Now concentrate on relaxing the muscles of the neck, imagining that the muscles are as floppy as a handful of rubber bands. Next, relax the muscles of the jaws, cheeks, and sides of the face. Relax the eyes, nose, forehead, and scalp.

Cleansing breath
Finally, take a long, slow, deep breath to eliminate tension that may remain.

Yoga

One of the oldest known health practices, yoga (which means *union* in Sanskrit) is the integration of physical, mental, and spiritual energies to promote health and wellness. The basic components of yoga include proper breathing, movement, and posture. While practicing specific postures, the practitioner pays close attention to his breathing, exhaling at certain times and inhaling at others. The breathing techniques are believed to promote relaxation and enhance the vital flow of energy known as *prana*.

 Numerous scientific studies have shown that the regular practice of yoga can produce the same physiologic changes as meditation. Known as the relaxation response, these changes include decreased heart and respiratory rates, improved cardiac and respiratory function, decreased blood pressure, decreased oxygen consumption, increased alpha wave activity, and EEG synchronicity, a change in brain wave activity occurring only in deep meditation.

Tai chi chuan

A form of exercise built on the mind-body connection, tai chi chuan (or tai chi) combines physical movement, meditation, and breathing to induce relaxation and improve balance, posture, coordination, endurance, strength, and flexibility. Tai chi also benefits patients who suffer from anxiety, stress, restlessness, and depression. Tai chi can be practiced by people of all ages, sizes, and physical abilities because it relies more on technique than strength. Participants perform a series of rhythmic movement patterns slowly and methodically.

Imagery

In imagery, patients use their imagination to promote relaxation, relieve symptoms (or better cope with them), and heal disease. Imagery is based on the principle that the mind and body are interconnected and can work together to encourage healing. Imagery can lower blood pressure and decrease heart rate. It can also affect brain wave activity, oxygen supply to the tissues, vascular constriction, skin temperatures, cochlear and pupillary reflexes, galvanic skin responses, salivation, and GI activity. According to imagery advocates, people with strong imaginations, including those who can literally worry themselves sick, are excellent candidates for using imagery.

Meditation

Meditation reduces stress, which in turn results in decreased oxygen consumption, heart rate, and respiratory rate, and also leads to improved mood and a feeling of calmness. The most common form of meditation, called concentrative meditation, involves focusing on an object to eliminate distractions in the mind. The focus in a meditative exercise may be a repetitive sound (such as a word, phrase, or simple musical tune), a peaceful imaginary scenario, or the body itself, as in concentrated deep rhythmic breathing. (See *Relaxation breathing.*) The focus may also

Advice from the experts

Relaxation breathing

Relaxation breathing can increase the lung capacity from 15% normally to around 80% during the exercise. With daily practice, relaxation breathing and the improvement in lung capacity that comes with it can become automatic.

Inhale

To practice relaxation breathing, inhale through your nose, but don't expand your chest. If your chest is expanding, you're breathing shallowly and actually constricting your lungs. When inhaling, your chest should remain unchanged, but you should expand your belly. Imagine there's a balloon in your stomach and your job is to blow as much air as possible into it.

Inhalation should take about 6 seconds. For comparison, people typically inhale for only about 2 seconds. Inhaling more slowly brings more oxygen into the lungs.

Pause and hold

After inhaling, pause and hold your breath for a few seconds. Pausing exercises your diaphragm and internal muscles. When you first start doing relaxation breathing, you may feel a little out of breath from the pausing. If you feel uncomfortable, you can skip the pauses for now and insert them when you've become more comfortable with the basic pattern of inhaling and exhaling.

Exhale

Next, exhale slowly and evenly for 6 seconds by relaxing the abdomen and allowing the lungs to expel the air. The chest may expand slightly at this point.

Be aware that when you're practicing relaxation breathing as a conscious exercise, you should breathe through your mouth gently, not forcefully. When breathing this way during normal activity, exhale through your nose.

Putting it all together

Using this breathing technique, take ten full, deep breaths. Inhale for 6 seconds, and then exhale for 6 seconds in a steady rhythm. After you learn the technique, there shouldn't be any pauses between inhalation and exhalation. If you have trouble with a 6-second cycle, find a cycle that's comfortable for you, such as a 3-second cycle, and gradually work your way up to 6 seconds.

Set aside 5 minutes three times a day to practice. If possible, practice your breathing while sitting comfortably in a chair with your feet flat on the floor and your arms resting loosely in your lap.

be a mantra, a word or phrase repeated over and over in a melodic rhythm.

Focusing on an object or thought of some kind prevents the undisciplined mind from flitting from subject to subject. As you grow in experience with meditation, you'll find it easier to prolong and sustain concentration.

Exercise your mind

Visualization

Visualization is similar to meditation except that in visualization you're guiding your thoughts toward a set of specific images. Visualization can take many forms, but a common one involves focusing on being in a quiet, safe place.

Setting

To perform visualization, go to a quiet area with as few distractions as possible. Sit comfortably in a chair, and take at least ten natural breaths. Close your eyes gently, and imagine the inside of your eyelids as a movie screen. Picture a physical setting that makes you feel calm and relaxed, such as a sunny clearing in the woods, a canoe ride on a still lake at sunrise, or a book-lined study with classical music playing in the background.

Colors and smells

Now sharpen your image of this place by using all of your senses to provide reality. See the flowers along the edge of the clearing. Feel the moisture in the morning mist. Listen to each note as the bassoons play off the sounds of the violins.

Sharpen the images with even more specific detail. What kind of trees are surrounding you? Are they old-growth or young trees? Is the clearing near a lake or stream? Can you hear the rushing water? Put as much detail as possible into your image.

Focus

As you work on the clarity of the vision, pay attention to your feelings. Focus on your sense of calm and restfulness. Let all the elements of the scene wash over your emotions. Remember your "place" when you finish your visualization session. When you visualize next, return to your place and add detail. Change its characteristics, if you like. Practice going to your quiet place on demand.

Another form of meditation involves "letting go" or "going with the flow" to become more sensitive to your environment. To do this, you need to be in a quiet, serene place, such as the shore, the woods, or a quiet place at home. Assume a comfortable position, such as the famous Lotus position or similar meditative pose. Take some deep breaths, relaxing your body a little each time you exhale.

Allow your thoughts to flow from one to the other without attempting to manipulate them. (See *Visualization*.) Allow your distractions to be played out in your mind until you can gently bring your attention back to a calm, peaceful state. The aim of this sort of meditation is to lose self-consciousness and not to think in the perspective of "I."

Caring for the mind

Nearly every cultural tradition contains techniques for promoting relaxation and reducing stress. You can turn your mind toward relaxation rather than stress and anxiety by controlling negative thoughts and building social supports.

Controlling negative thoughts

Some stress can be accentuated by imagining the worst possible scenario. The imagination can be highly creative. It can veer off in frightening directions if allowed to do so and create images and events that increase anxiety.

You've got to accentuate the positive...

Positive, creative imagery can have a suggestive effect that starts the mind moving toward a goal and weakens or overcomes negative images. By imagining what goals you want to reach and visualizing how you'll achieve each goal, you can replace negative thoughts with positive ones. (See *The power of positive thinking,* page 94.) If you imagine failure, you're more likely to fail; if you imagine success, you're more likely to succeed.

I'm accentuating the positive. I'm *positively* swamped!

...and eliminate the negative

To rid yourself of negative thoughts, find a quiet place, sit or lie down, close your eyes, and imagine your body as being two-dimensional with the interior completely dark. Slowly begin to inhale and exhale. Think of each exhalation as forcing some of the interior darkness from your body. Inhale and exhale the darkness until you feel that the interior of your body is no longer dark. You'll soon begin to feel the stress disappearing with each exhalation.

Another technique involves stopping yourself each time your inner voice says something negative. Replace these thoughts with positive thoughts or a mantra. You may have to repeat these thoughts several times until you conquer your anxiety, but gradually it may help you to eliminate angry or frightening thoughts.

Exercise your mind

The power of positive thinking

If you plan to succeed and visualize yourself succeeding, then you're more likely to ultimately succeed. Nurture your power of positive thinking by:

• "psyching" yourself up for important events. Think about the upcoming situation, and visualize it as being a successful experience.

• talking to yourself in a positive manner. Think of yourself as the little train that could. Repeat over and over, "I know I can. I know I can."

• preparing properly. Develop a plan of action as well as contingency or alternative plans in case circumstances change.

• labeling an upcoming event that could cause undue tension as a positive learning experience.

• looking at examinations and other potentially stressful events as opportunities to prove yourself by showing others what you know or what you can do. Avoid looking at these events as tests of what you don't know or can't do. Looking at them as positive opportunities can give you a feeling of power and accomplishment.

Building social supports

A strong social network can help control and improve a person's ability to respond effectively to stress. Social networks can take many forms, including:
• family
• friends
• peers at work
• fellow students
• religious groups
• people with shared interests, such as sports or hobbies.

These social supports give you an outlet for discussing problems with people who care for you and want to help you. Discussion of stress-producing problems can also give you new perspectives on chronic problems. Prayer can provide quiet time and help you focus priorities so you can better deal with stress-provoking situations.

> Use social supports in times of stress.

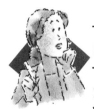

Quick quiz

1. The body's response to beneficial environmental stimuli is called:
- A. coherence.
- B. eustress.
- C. fight or flight.

Answer: B. The body's response to beneficial environmental stimuli is called eustress, which keeps us alert, motivates us to face challenges, and drives us to solve problems.

2. When faced with a stressor, people with a strong sense of coherence react:
- A. more positively to the stressor.
- B. more negatively to the stressor.
- C. highly intensely to the stressor.

Answer: A. People with a strong sense of coherence feel more in control of themselves and react more positively to stress than do people with a weaker sense of coherence.

3. The phase in the general adaptation syndrome (GAS) in which epinephrine is released from the adrenal glands is the phase called:
- A. reaction.
- B. resistance.
- C. exhaustion.

Answer: B. During the second phase of the GAS, resistance, the hormone epinephrine is released from the adrenal glands.

4. The form of exercise that combines physical movement, meditation, and breathing to induce relaxation is called:
- A. imagery.
- B. tai chi chuan.
- C. yoga.

Answer: B. A form of exercise built on the mind-body connection, tai chi chuan (or tai chi) combines physical movement, meditation, and breathing to induce relaxation and improve balance, posture, coordination, endurance, strength, and flexibility.

Scoring

☆☆☆   If you answered all four questions correctly, wowsa, wowsa, wowsa! You're our Stress Manager extraordinaire!

☆☆   If you answered three questions correctly, fabulous! You're clearly not one to freeze and forget!

☆   If you answered fewer than three questions correctly, don't be glum. Just repeat this mantra to get back on track: "You stress, I stress, we *all* stress for eustress!"

Reading and classroom strategies

Just the facts

In this chapter, you'll learn:

♦ why effective reading skills are critical for success in studying and how they can be improved with the consistent application of basic reading strategies

♦ how to prepare for a lecture ahead of time and why you should review your notes afterward

♦ why using the principles of active reading and listening can improve comprehension.

Reading skills

Students receive more than 75% of their course information from printed materials. Solid reading skills, then, are essential for successful studying. Effective reading skills involve strategies to improve comprehension as well as reading speed.

Comprehension techniques

Reading and understanding course material provides support for lectures and classroom activities and leads to a thorough understanding of the topic under study. Improving reading comprehension involves skimming for ideas, using active reading skills, and summarizing the material.

Skimming for ideas

The first step in reading a chapter in a textbook is to look the chapter over without trying to read every word. Skimming the chapter gives you an idea of the content and shows you how the material is organized. By thinking about the structure before actually reading the material, your brain can organize the learning to come, which improves your ability to understand the content and recall information in the chapter.

Getting to know you

Before reading a chapter in detail, look at the illustrations and read the captions. Then read the introductory paragraph and all the headings in the chapter. Finally, read the chapter summary.

Use the same skimming techniques to read an entire book. First, look at the title page. Read about the author on the book jacket or the *About the Author* page. Read the preface or other introductory material. Examine the table of contents to obtain a better idea about its content. Review the pages, noting especially emphasized words in bold or italics. Finally, read vocabulary or glossary terms listed at the beginning or end of the chapter as appropriate.

A picture is worth a thousand words

Review all graphs, charts, tables, and illustrations. These supplemental content are intended to expand on or clarify the material covered in the main text, so use them to your advantage.

Getting ready to read

Reading comprehension is enhanced when the reading material is relevant to your own background. For example, an experienced X-ray technician could most likely read faster and more readily understand a chapter about the advantages of using contrast medium in certain procedures. The technician's background gives her a knowledge of relevant vocabulary and an ability to more quickly comprehend connections among concepts. As a result, she can more easily comprehend the material. (See *Improving your reading comprehension*.)

To more easily understand material about a complex topic, try reading less advanced material on the same subject, listening to a lecture on it, or attending a seminar on a related topic.

Improving your reading comprehension

Improving your reading comprehension doesn't have to be an impossible dream. Following these guidelines can help you more readily comprehend every reading assignment you have:

• Keep your purpose for reading squarely in mind.

• If the main idea is unstated, identify the topic by looking for repetitions of key words or phrases.

• Retrieve the background knowledge necessary to understand the text, including looking up unknown words and referring to less advanced resources.

• Restate the main idea through paraphrasing, summarizing, or synthesizing.

There's a pattern here

Understanding how the text itself is organized can help you focus on the most important parts of the text. Common structural components include:

• subject development or definition text structure, which identifies a concept and lists its supporting details. These paragraphs are usually found at the beginning of major sections.

• enumeration or sequence text, in which major points are listed by number or in sequence and are commonly preceded by such clue words as *first, second, next, then,* and others.

• compare-and-contrast text, which expresses relationships between two or more ideas. Comparisons show how ideas are similar; contrasting statements show how they're different.

• cause-and-effect text, which shows how one idea or event results from another idea or event.

Active reading

Reading actively fosters comprehension by involving more than one sense. To become a more active reader, you can:

• Read out loud.

• Take notes on the material you read.

• Formulate some questions you'd like answered while you read.

• Think about the important points as outlined by the table of contents.

• Avoid arguing with the author when reading (analyzing the text can be done later).
• Mark areas you'd like to read again.

Read at your best

Read during part of the day when you feel comfortable, alert, and unhurried. If you know you have to read 25 pages today and that you get sleepy after lunch, avoid trying to complete your reading after lunch. Choose a time when you're feeling more alert. Likewise, don't try to do too much reading at once. If you've been reading for a long time and begin to feel your concentration slipping, take a 5-minute break.

Staying distraction-free

Watching television, listening to music with lyrics, and engaging in numerous otherwise enjoyable activities can be distracting when trying to study. Avoid distractions by finding a quiet place to read. Sit at a desk or in a straight-backed chair bathed in natural or incandescent lighting. Try to avoid getting too comfortable and, as a result, becoming sleepy. Have a healthy snack, and keep water handy to stave off hunger and thirst.

Have a highlighter handy

If you own the book you're reading, use a highlighter to mark important ideas. (See *Power-reading symbols.*) If you don't own the book, use colored sticky notes for marking key areas. In either case, don't overdo it. Marking up too much material makes the material meaningless after a while. When buying a used text, never choose one that has already been highlighted or otherwise marked up by another student.

Keep these tips in mind when highlighting:
• If you skimmed the material before reading it, use your marks to note details that provide answers to your questions.
• Mark material you believe the instructor considers most important.
• Consider the difficulty of the language when deciding what content to mark. (See *Marking and labeling text,* page 102.) Subject depth, the number of details given, and overall vocabulary affect how much you understand.

Keep in mind that highlighters and sticky notes are indexing tools; they can help you find information but they

Advice from the experts

Power-reading symbols

Using shortcuts for labeling text can help you read faster while still understanding the text. This table shows commonly used symbols for labeling text.

Symbol	Meaning
ex	example or experiment
form	formula
MI	main idea
! or *	important information
→	results, leads to, steps in a sequence
(1), (2), (3)	label important points
circled word	summarizes process
?	disagree or unclear
term	important term
summ	summary
{}	indicates that certain pieces of information relate
opin	author's opinion, rather than fact
∴	therefore

can do nothing about helping you *learn* the information. Whenever you mark a section of your book, be sure to do something with it later, such as writing a summary of highlighted information or drawing a chart or diagram to summarize the information.

Label main ideas

Every chapter has a central premise, and every paragraph within that chapter presents at least one main idea. The main ideas and supporting details of each paragraph support the central premise of the chapter.

In a typical paragraph, the topic sentence tells you the main idea. The topic sentence usually appears at the beginning or end of the paragraph but may appear anywhere. Pay particular attention to topic sentences, highlighting the sentence or parts of the sentence as appropriate.

So what you're saying is...

Take notes while you read. If you can rephrase the material, then you probably understand it. Comprehension

Advice from the experts

Marking and labeling text

Marking and labeling text can help you retain knowledge about the reading you've done and make later reference easier. Keep these points in mind when marking and labeling text.

- Read a paragraph or section completely before marking anything.
- Mark points that answer questions you might have had before reading.
- Number lists, reasons, or other items that occur in a series or sequence.
- Identify important terms, dates, places, and names.
- Write main idea summaries, questions, and other comments in the margins.
- Put a question mark beside unclear or confusing information.
- Put a star or exclamation point beside information your instructor emphasizes in class, possible test questions, or what seems to be extremely important information.
- Write comments on the table of contents or make your own table of contents of important topics inside the front cover of the book or on the title page.

builds on itself. Some concepts (in math, for example) must be understood before you can move on. One method of note taking while you read involves drawing graphics of the material. Graphics are sometimes more memorable than words.

Getting personal

The active reader assimilates information to relate to her own experience, thus making the information more easily remembered because it's more personal. The more personal the information, the more meaningful the material. Make the material more meaningful by:

- making associations of personal relevance. For example, perhaps an important date can be associated with a birth date.
- allowing it to evoke an emotional response. A deep emotional response to information or even something that strikes you funny can make the information more interesting and therefore more entrenched in memory.
- taking advantage of your brain's ability to recall pictures, graphics, and illustrations. Draw out what you learn. Make patterns, doodles, and drawings that make sense to you.

Criticism counts

Read critically, asking yourself questions about the text. Question the authority of the author or the reliability of the information provided. Questioning the content forces you to think critically about the information, which may open doors to greater understanding of the content and improve retention. Here are examples of critical questions:

• How can I apply this information with a patient?
• How does this information relate to what I studied last week?
• Does the information validate ideas in other resources or contradict other reading?
• Under what circumstances were the data collected?
• How was the information verified?
• Do inconsistencies exist in the information?
• How does the author answer his own questions?
• Has the author made any assumptions?
• Are the author's statements based on knowledge, facts, experiences, or opinions?
• Is the author being objective?
• Do I disagree with the author? Why?
• If I was playing "devil's advocate," what questions would I ask the author? What examples would I include that the author didn't?
• What do I want to know that the author hasn't told me?

Look it up

If you come across a word you've never seen, don't understand, or can't pronounce, look it up in a dictionary. First, though, try to derive the meaning of the word from its context in the sentence and from its root words, prefixes, and suffixes. Try to pronounce it. Then read the dictionary meaning and pronunciation of the word, noting both in the margin of your notes. Keep in mind that if the author used the word once, he'll probably use it again.

If the text contains a lot of difficult words, you may want to read through some of the material first, marking the difficult words or making a list of the words that need to be looked up. Then go back for a second pass with a dictionary close at hand.

It's especially important to understand the meaning of technical words when reading scientific material. Technical terms are integral to understanding scientific

> When you can anticipate the reading and you know where it's going, you've become an active reader. Congratulations!

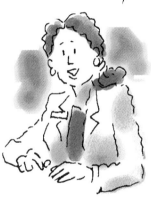

principles being discussed. By building your vocabulary, you not only understand the material better but you also become better able to express yourself, both in written form and verbally.

Summarize the material

In general, textbooks use the same method in every chapter to summarize the chapter's content. This information may be contained in a summary paragraph or a group of summary questions. After reading your assignment, look at the chapter summary and table of contents again to be sure you understood the material in the format intended by the author. If there is an area you're unsure of, read through that information again or ask for clarification from your instructor, who can probably explain it better.

If you need to read the material again to understand it better, do it differently the second time. Read the material more slowly, perhaps, concentrating on one sentence at a time. Or, read the material aloud. Make sure you understand each sentence before moving to the next. Try to relate the new idea to what the author has already covered.

Use what you know

After you've finished the assignment, find ways to apply your newly found knowledge, even if just by talking about it. Share what you read with others. Talking about the material reflects your ability to restate what you've learned, which reinforces your comprehension.

Increasing your reading rate

The average college student reads fiction and nontechnical materials at a rate between 250 and 350 words per minute. To reach peak efficiency in reading, experts say your reading speed should approach 500 to 700 words per minute. Some people can read 1,000 words per minute or even faster.

Increasing the rate at which you read can help you move through assignments more quickly, thus improving your study efficiency. However, keep in mind that when it comes to reading speed, faster is not better if you don't understand what you've read. The trick is to read faster *and* comprehend the material.

Rapid eye movement

The key to rapid reading is to sweep your eyes from left to right across the page, making as few stops — called fixations — as possible. Readers who can see a full phrase at a time can read faster than one who sees one word at a time.

When you read, your eyes tend to jump toward information you've already read. In some situations, you can spend as much as 90% of your reading time with your eyes looking away from what you think you're looking at. Training your eyes to reduce eye movement can double reading speed almost immediately.

Retraining your eyes

To train your eyes to stay where you want them when reading, hold a blank index card above each line you read. As you progress down the page, cover each line with the card after you've finished reading it. At first, you might find this process physically different because your eyes naturally want to scan back up the page, but after a few weeks, you'll find that you're reading faster than ever.

Role of speed in the reading process

Does reading faster compromise comprehension? Researchers say no, particularly if the technique used to improve the reading rate focuses on improving basic reading habits. Most adults are able to increase their rate of reading without lowering comprehension. In fact, an increase in rate is typically paralleled by an increase in comprehension. Furthermore, people who increase their reading speed won't understand material better if they reduce their reading rate. So, reading faster is, in many instances, a win-win situation.

What's slowing you down?

A number of factors play a role in keeping the reading rate slower than it could be, including:
• reading word by word
• slow reaction time
• slow recognition and response to the material
• reading out loud
• faulty eye movements, including wrong placement on the page, faulty return sweep, and irregular rhythm and movement

- habitual rereading
- inattention
- impaired retention
- lack of practice
- deliberate rate suppression out of fear of losing comprehension
- habitual slow reading
- poor differentiation of which aspects are important and which can be swept over
- inability to remember critical details.

Before you increase your reading rate

Certain conditions should be met before trying to increase your reading rate, including:

- Have your eyes checked. Slow reading is sometimes related to uncorrected vision defects. To ease eye strain and lessen eye movement while reading, hold your book 4" to 6" farther away from your eyes than you normally do. Be sure to hold reading material at least 15" away from your eyes.
- Avoid sounding out words as you read. Reading silently is 2 to 3 times faster than reading aloud. Concentrate on key words and ideas rather than on whispering each word to yourself.
- Avoid rereading. Rereading is generally just a bad habit rather than a need to improve comprehension. Many of the ideas that may need further explanation are explained later in the text. Slower readers tend to reread more often, possibly due to an inability to concentrate or a lack of confidence in the ability to comprehend the material.
- Develop a wider eye span by focusing on taking in more words on a line as you read. (See *Widening your eye span.*) Most people read one word at a time, but the brain can assimilate several words at once. Developing a wider eye span helps you read reduce the number of reading stops, which, in turn, yields a faster reading rate.

Rate adjustment

Your reading rate shouldn't be the same for all the material you read. Adjust your reading rate according to the difficulty level and the specific purpose for reading. Use a faster rate for easy, familiar, or interesting material and a slower rate for unfamiliar content or language. (See *Calculating average reading speed,* page 108.) Keep in mind that,

Exercise your mind

Widening your eye span

Readers whose eyes take in more than one word at a time can read faster and retain just as much as a reader whose eyes take in only one word at a time. Try this exercise to help you see the whole page rather than zooming in on single words. Perform this exercise 5 minutes a day every day for several weeks. Use a large book when practicing.

1. Flip through the pages of the book quickly, turning them from the top with your left hand and scrolling left-to-right down each page with the edge of your right hand.

2. Follow your right hand down each page with your eyes, trying to see as many words as possible. Start by drifting down each page for 2 or 3 seconds, gradually reducing the time spent on each page until you can go as fast as you can turn pages.

3. Start by reading at a rate of 20 pages per minute. Slowly increase this rate over a period of 1 to 2 months to as many as 100 pages per minute.

as your vocabulary improves, so does your reading speed. The fewer stops you make to stumble over an unknown word, the faster you can move through the material.

What's your purpose?

Avoid planning to read your assignments at your maximum reading rate. Take into account those areas of the reading assignment that may be difficult to read as well as those that may be easier. Decide on your purpose in reading, and then read at a rate that best provides the level of comprehension you require.

Know when to slow down...

In general, you should slow your reading speed when you encounter:
• complex sentence or paragraph structure
• material that must be remembered in detail
• detailed or highly technical material, including complicated directions and statements of difficult principles
• unfamiliar or unclear terminology. Try to understand the material in context, and then continue reading, returning to that section later.
• unfamiliar or abstract concepts. Try to internalize the information by making it applicable to your personal life.

Advice from the experts

Calculating average reading speed

Use your average reading rate when planning your reading schedule. To figure your average reading rate, perform this calculation:

• Count the total number of words in 10 lines of text. Divide this figure by 10 to get the average number of words per line.

• Count the total number of lines on a full page of text.

• Multiply the average number of words per line by the number of lines on a page. This is the word density of the material. Keep in mind that word density can vary from book to book.

• Timing yourself, read for exactly 10 minutes.

• Multiply the number of pages read in 10 minutes by the word density to get an approximate number of words read.

• Divide the total number of words read by 10, the number of minutes read. This is your reading rate for this text.

Sample calculation

Here's a sample calculation of a person's average reading speed for a textbook that consists of about 125 words in 10 lines and holds 52 lines on each page.

$$\frac{125 \text{ words}}{10 \text{ lines}} = 12.5 \text{ words/line}$$

$$52 \text{ lines/page} \times 12.5 \text{ words/line} = 650 \text{ words/page}$$

$$\frac{650 \text{ words/page} \times 3.5 \text{ pages read in 10 minutes}}{10 \text{ minutes}} = 227.5 \text{ words/minute}$$

...and when to speed up

In general, accelerate your reading speed when you encounter:

• simple material that contains few new ideas

• broad or generalized ideas or statements of ideas already explained

• detailed explanations and elaborations of ideas that aren't necessary for your purpose

• examples and illustrations that cover material you already understand. Examples and illustrations are included in the text to clarify ideas, but they become unnecessary if you already know the material.

No stopping

Of the more than 600,000 words in the English language, 400 of them are used over and over again in most of the material you'll ever read. These 400 words, called structure words, make up 65% of printed works. Structure words include such words as *the, and, to, from, but, however,* and similar basic words. Even though you shouldn't completely skip words in a sentence, you shouldn't stop on structure words either. Let your eye take them in along with neighboring words to speed reading along.

Practice, practice, practice

As you practice reading faster, you become more adept at it. However, always read all of the words in a passage; otherwise, you may misinterpret the author's meaning or miss a relevant point. In addition, reading faster than you can understand the material can provoke frustration and anxiety.

You might be concerned that if you go faster, you'll miss words. As with any skill, practice makes perfect — or at least better. You may also find it helpful to visualize yourself as an improved, faster reader. Visualizing yourself as you would like to be can help you attain your goal.

Basic classroom skills

The instructor's goal in giving a lecture is to make the content easier to understand. The instructor includes explanations and clarifies ideas and information included in your textbook. To improve your ability to retain information provided in the classroom, you'll need to take specific steps before and during class and to organize your notes and other class materials for maximum efficiency.

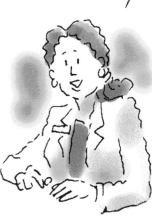

As you prepare for class, jot down questions that come to mind.

Preparations for class

To prepare properly for a lecture, look at the reading assignment and read the section headings. Then look at charts or illustrations in the chapter, and read the caption for each. Skim the main text to identify basic concepts and the most important information.

Look for words emphasized in bold or italics print. At this point, your goal is to gain a general understanding of the content. Try not to get bogged down in difficult sections; the lecture may clarify those sections for you.

Write questions that come to mind as you read, but keep the questions brief — most of them will probably be answered during the lecture. If they aren't, you'll be better prepared to ask the instructor for clarification.

Another quick review

After you finish your first reading, look again at the headings and illustrations. This quick review increases your long-term memory and allows you to more effectively integrate what you learn in class with what you read before class.

Tips during class

During class, pay special attention to:
- contents of handouts
- anything written on the chalkboard
- anything the instructor stresses or repeats
- your instructor's response to questions from classmates
- your own thoughts, questions, or reactions to lecture material
- anything the instructor takes a long time to explain
- anything discussed that isn't covered in the textbook, particularly the instructor's personal views
- how the instructor presents the information in class — for instance, whether he presents the "big picture" or the details
- the beginning and end of the lecture. Instructors often summarize their entire lecture during the first few minutes and, in the last few minutes, summarize major points and other important points there wasn't time to cover.

If it's important enough for the instructor to write on the board, remember it!

Classroom communication

In a lecture, communication takes place primarily between the instructor and the students. How well you listen to your instructor depends on your background knowledge, the difficulty of the concepts being covered, and your purpose in listening. (See *Levels of listening*, page 112.) For most students, listening to lectures is a passive activity but it doesn't have to be. Try to stay involved in the lecture, thinking of questions as the speaker lectures. Jot down a key word or two about the question in the margin of your notes. Then, when the instructor asks if anyone has questions, refer to your notes to ask the questions you raised earlier.

When you get too much, too fast

When the instructor seems to run through a lecture quickly, covering a lot of material in a limited time, it may be wise to interrupt and ask for clarification, particularly if you familiarized yourself with the material beforehand but still don't understand it. When asking for clarification, be as specific as possible. Try to show that you understood some of what was said by rephrasing the information in your own words.

Talking...too...slowly

Daydreaming is more likely to be a problem when a class is slow. To stave off boredom and loss of concentration, try to rephrase, repeat, and apply what's been said. Use slow parts of the class to review material in your head. Review concepts and definitions that your instructor has introduced and try rephrasing them in your own words. Then repeat new phrases and definitions to yourself and try to memorize them. Or, try to anticipate your instructor's next move. This keeps you involved in the class and trains you to follow your instructor's thought processes, which helps you to perform better on assignments.

In too deep?

If you're not understanding the material well, you might not have the background that other students in the class have. The feeling of being lost usually comes from the lack of a sufficient foundation of knowledge in a particular area. In each class, the instructor assumes a certain amount of knowledge on the part of the student and tries to build on that knowledge.

If that foundation doesn't exist, it's easy to tune out what the instructor is saying. Instead of tuning out the instructor, focus on tuning in even more carefully. Keep taking notes even though you don't understand everything. Jot down words and phrases that you don't understand. Look them up right after the class or ask your instructor for clarification.

Keeping the lines open

Maintaining communication between you and your instructor can help your instructor clarify points of misun-

Levels of listening

Listening involves several levels, depending on the effort expended by the listener. This chart describes the different levels of listening.

Level	Description
Reception	hearing without thought
Attention	listening passively; no effort to understand what's being said
Definition	lowest level of active listening; giving meaning to isolated facts and details; no overall organizational plan
Integration	relating new information to old learning
Interpretation	synthesizing information; putting information into own words
Implication	drawing conclusions
Application	applying information to personal experience; using information in new situations
Evaluation	judging information in terms of accuracy and relevance

derstanding. In addition, your feedback can help reinforce the instructor's method or point out where a lecture might be weak.

Coping with ineffective lecturers

You might need to compensate for a less effective speaker by defining, integrating, and interpreting information and drawing conclusions for yourself. (See *Compensating for an ineffective lecturer.*) Finding ways to apply information and judging its value then becomes one of your primary jobs.

In a lecture, the speaker controls what information is conveyed to the class. Your job is to determine what the instructor expects and to keep that purpose in mind while listening and reacting to the lecture. To help you maintain active listening during a lecture:

• Keep your purpose for listening in mind.
• Pay careful attention to the instructor's introductory and summary statements, which usually state main points.
• Continue to take notes.
• Sit comfortably erect to convey your interest and stave off sleepiness.
• Keep your eyes on the instructor.

Advice from the experts

Compensating for an ineffective lecturer

Your main task when faced with any lecturer is to get the most out of the class regardless of the effectiveness of the lecturer. When a lecturer isn't effective, you can still obtain the knowledge you need by following a few guidelines. This chart explains what to do when an instructor falls short of expectations.

If your instructor fails to do this	Then you do this
Explain goals of the lecture	Use your text and syllabus to set objectives.
Review previous lecture material before beginning a new lecture	Set aside time before each class to review notes.
State main ideas in an introduction and summary of the lecture	Write short summaries of the day's lecture immediately after class.
Provide an outline of the lecture	Preview assigned readings before class, or outline notes after class.
Provide "wait time" for writing notes	Politely ask the instructor to repeat information or speak more slowly.
Speak clearly with appropriate volume	Politely ask the instructor to repeat information or speak more loudly, or move closer to him.
Answer questions without sarcasm	Refrain from taking comments personally.
Stay on topic	Discover how anecdotes relate to the topic, or use anecdotes as a memory cue.
Refrain from reading directly from the text	Mark passages in text as the instructor reads, or summarize or outline these passages in the text margin.
Emphasize main points	Supplement lectures through text previews and reading.
Use transition words	Ask the instructor for a clarifying example, discuss idea with other students, or create an example yourself.
Give examples to illustrate difficult ideas	Supplement notes with terms listed in the text, and highlight information contained in the lecture.
Write important words, dates, and other key information on the chalkboard	Use the text glossary or a dictionary.
Define important terms	Relate information to what you know about the topic, or create a clarifying example for yourself.

- Concentrate on what the instructor is saying to ignore external distractions and eliminate internal ones.
- Question the material.
- Listen for transition words that signal main points.
- Mark words or references you don't understand for later investigation.
- Adjust your listening and note-taking pace to the lecture.

• Avoid being a distraction yourself by sitting still and staying silent.

Active listening

Active listening occurs when you consciously think about how you're listening and use strategies to improve and maximize your listening skills. To improve your active listening skills, you need to:
• Avoid behaviors that can interfere with listening.
• Recognize main ideas.
• Use transition cues effectively.
• Differentiate more important information from less important information.

Avoid interfering behaviors

A number of behaviors can interfere with your understanding when listening to a lecturer or other speaker, including:
• allowing distractions to interfere with listening
• avoiding difficult material
• becoming overexcited by something in the lecture
• considering the subject uninteresting
• criticizing the speaker's delivery or mannerisms
• daydreaming
• faking attentiveness
• letting emotion-laden words arouse personal antagonism
• listening primarily for facts instead of ideas
• trying to outline everything.

Recognizing main ideas

Every lecture is structured to center around main ideas. This structure leads to certain patterns that vary with the instructor's purposes. Be aware that in a lecture an instructor may:
• introduce new topics or summarize information
• list or rank details
• present opposing sides of an issue
• identify causes and effects or problems and solutions
• discuss concepts using supporting details.

Anticipating through transition clues

Signal words and other verbal markers help you identify and anticipate the flow of a lecture. Becoming familiar with transition words helps you organize lecture notes and listen more actively. For example, the word *conversely* probably indicates that the lecturer is about to present an opposing point of view. *Therefore* means the lecturer is summing up cause and effect. *Finally* means the instructor is getting to the end of his point or series of points.

> Ahh, the word "finally." He must be getting to the end. Whew!

Identifying important information

The ability to identify important information contributes to your ability to become a more active listener. Although instructors emphasize main points differently, they have similar ways of conveying important information. Some instructors, for instance, write key information on the chalkboard. Others outline the entire lecture on the chalkboard before class begins. Some write key points or terms on the board as they lecture.

Copying outlines or lists of terms from the chalkboard aids learning in three ways. First, you learn as you write. Copying the outline also provides a nutshell view of the lecture's content and serves as a guide for study later.

Instructors also convey information by:
- pausing, which gives you more time to take comprehensive notes
- repeating information
- changing the tone or volume of his voice to make a point
- telling the class what's worth remembering for a test
- using body language. If your instructor gestures to stress a point, it's often an essential point for you to understand.
- using visual aids. The use of films, overhead transparencies, videotapes, and other audiovisual materials signals important topics.
- referring to specific text pages. Information an instructor knows by page number is worth noting and remembering.

Learn the LISAN method

Active listening is the key to taking notes during a lecture. The LISAN method of taking notes encourages active listening and can improve understanding and retention. The LISAN method involves these guidelines:
- **Lead**, don't follow. Anticipate what the instructor is going to say.
- **Ideas**. What's the main idea?

• **S**ignal words. Listen for words that tell you the direction the instructor is taking.
• **A**ctively listen. Ask questions, be prepared.
• **N**ote taking. Write down key points. Be selective.

Developing learning skills

You can also develop your learning skills as you listen. Development of these skills involves memorization, applying knowledge, interpreting information, and recognizing shifts in teaching styles.

Is it live, or memorized?

Introductory courses tend to demand a lot of memorization. Stay alert for information you should commit to memory. Items such as phrases, dates, and diagrams written on a chalkboard are probably items that the instructor expects you to remember. If the instructor takes the time to write a definition or prepare a handout or slide, that means the information is important and should be remembered. If the instructor speaks more slowly than usual or repeats information, he's probably giving you time to take notes on the material.

How canst I apply it? Let me count the ways

Many instructors arrange their classes and assignments to encourage you to apply the information they provide to clinical situations. Pay attention to how the instructor structures the class. For instance, if the instructor gives written assignments on the material, you'll need to show in writing how well you can apply your new knowledge.

Does the instructor spend class time working through problems or cases? Then you'll probably be expected to know how to work through such problems on a test. Does the instructor ask students to solve problems at the chalkboard? If so, expect to be asked to demonstrate your new knowledge to your peers.

Hmmm, how should I interpret that?

Many advanced science and health classes require that students use their interpretative skills. The instructor tries to foster development of those skills by asking a lot of general questions and offering guidance. In these kinds of classes, the students do most of the talking, however, and the assignments tend to consist primarily of reading and observing.

Shifts in teaching styles

Be on the lookout for shifts in teaching style. For example, if an instructor stops a class discussion to write dates on the chalkboard, then he has switched from an interpretive mode to a memorization mode. Write down the dates. Some instructors give obvious clues to what's important to study, even by saying something as clear and simple as, "This is important."

Other clues aren't as obvious. Look for patterns in your instructor's behavior such as the instructor's getting up and pacing whenever he begins warming up to an important point. The more attuned you are to the instructor's behaviors, the more knowledge you can gain from the material being presented.

Organizing lecture content

Lectures can be text-dependent, meaning that they follow the organization of the text closely, or text-independent, in which other media are used to enhance the delivery of information.

Lectures by the book

During a text-dependent lecture, write notes and instructions emphasized during the lecture directly in your textbook, highlighting or underlining as the instructor speaks. This is an especially helpful technique if you read the text before class. You can also cross out information your instructor says is unnecessary and note important information in the margins of the chapter and in your notebook.

Working without backup

When lectures are independent of the text, they're based on what the instructor thinks is most important about the topic. In those instances, your responsibility for taking notes increases. Because you don't have the text to use as a backup source, review or outline the lecture soon after class to give it some form of organization. Discuss your notes with other students or augment the lecture with supplemental reading. Set some

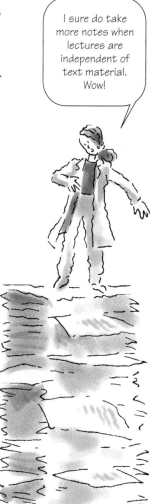

I sure do take more notes when lectures are independent of text material. Wow!

study objectives to help you create a purpose for learning and increase your recall.

Stimulating the senses

Instructors use a variety of media — handouts, films, slides, models, and so on — to stimulate your senses during lectures. Media offer visually interesting ways to add knowledge and information, arouse emotion or interest, or increase skills and performance.

When an instructor creates or chooses the medium to be used, the information it contains tends to be course-specific and corresponds closely to what your instructor expects you to know. Your responsibility is to recognize your instructor's purposes for using each particular medium and judge its worth in meeting your learning needs. For example, if you have extensive knowledge of a topic, a film about that topic may serve only as a review. If the topic is new to you, the same film may be aimed at building background knowledge.

Student-teacher conferences

Whenever you have questions about the content discussed in class, the instructor's expectations of you as a learner, or other important aspects of a course, you might want to set up a conference with the instructor. Before the conference, make sure you have a specific topic of discussion. Your first test might make an ideal subject, particularly if you feel as if you're struggling with the course material.

Having a conference with your instructor also helps you understand the instructor better and to demonstrate your interest in improving your performance. Even if you think you're doing well in a class, meeting with the instructor can help ensure that your perception is accurate as well as establish rapport.

Effective note-taking skills

Taking notes may be the most crucial part of active listening during lecture. In your effort to capture everything of significance said by the instructor, you'll not only need to use all of your listening ability and concentration during the lecture but also have a good system for recording what was said. Taking effective notes involves understanding why you take notes in the first place and following some practical guidelines for note taking.

Usefulness of notes

Notes often trigger your memory of the lecture or the text. In general, students who review notes achieve more than those who don't. Researchers have found that if important information was contained in notes, students tended to remember that information 34% of the time. Information not found in notes was remembered only 5% of the time. Even if you understand your instructor's lecture fully and have no questions, take notes anyway. Later, you'll want to know what the instructor thought was important, and you'll use the notes to refresh your memory.

Listen up!

Taking notes also makes you pay more attention to the new material, thereby allowing you to become more familiar with it. Note taking requires more effort than reading, and therefore requires you to take an active role in class. By paraphrasing and condensing information as you take notes, you show your understanding of the information and your ability to relate the information to your background knowledge.

Tips for taking notes

To take effective notes, you'll need to use your own form of note-taking shorthand, organize your notes after class, keep your notes personal, avoid using a tape recorder, and employ other note-taking strategies.

Shrthnd spds note tkng

Taking notes rapidly involves doing as little writing as possible while capturing all of the facts, principles, and ideas expressed by the lecturer. Fast note taking can be enhanced by:
• abbreviating common words consistently (see *Common note-taking abbreviations and symbols*)
• leaving out conjunctions, prepositions, and other words not essential to understanding the thought
• thinking before you write (but without thinking so long that you fall behind)

Advice from the experts

Common note-taking abbreviations and symbols

To speed note taking, get in the habit of using abbreviations and symbols. This chart lists common abbreviations and symbols used for taking notes.

Abbreviations		Symbols	
abt	about	®	right
b/c	because	Ⓛ	left
dx	diagnose or diagnosis	↑	increase, increased, or increasing
e.g.	for example	↓	decrease, decreased, or decreasing
h/a	headache	→	leads to or causes
hx	history	>	more than
imp	important	<	less than
incl	including	Δ	change
pt	patient	~	about, approximately
px	physical	+	and, in addition
rx	treat or treatment	#	pounds or number
s/e	side effects	☆	important or stressed by instructor
s/s	signs and symptoms	p̄	after
w/	with	ā	before
w/o	without	–	negative
		c̄	with
		s̄	without

• creating a shorthand word or symbol for something used repeatedly in a lecture — for example, abbreviating systolic blood pressure as SBP in a discussion about hypertension
• marking for emphasis, such as through the use of asterisks, exclamation points, underlining, color coding, or highlighting
• using shapes or varying handwriting sizes to stay organized. You're more likely to recall information supplemented with visual clues, such as geometric shapes or different-sized handwriting.

Postclass organization

After class, organize your notes. Write down the date at the beginning of each lecture, and number the pages so you can keep track of what you're doing. Make a note of your assignments, what they involve, and when they're due.

Keep 'em personal

The most effective notes are personal, reflecting the background knowledge and understanding of the person who takes them. Borrowed or bought notes require no effort or action on the part of the learner and so do little to help the student learn. To get the most out of notes for a class, be sure you attend the class yourself and take your own notes.

Borrowed notes do have a place, however, when they're all that's available. If you've been absent from class, you might have no choice but to borrow someone's notes.

Nix on the tape recorder

Tape recording a lecture can be useful but only if you also take notes during the lecture, allowing the taped material to pick up any important points you miss. Otherwise, using a tape recorder to record lectures is probably not a good idea. Here's why:

• Listening to the tape takes as long as, if not longer than, the lecture itself.

• To record the main ideas and highlights of the lecture, you have to make notes from the tape, which takes even longer.

• Taped material doesn't reflect diagrams or additional written material the instructor may have used during the class.

• Technical difficulties, such as a flawed tape or a dead battery, sometimes arise, causing you to miss part or all of a lecture.

• Some instructors may not allow the use of tape recorders. Ask the instructor before class whether it's permissible to record a lecture.

If you're unable to attend a class, however, asking a classmate to audiotape the class may prove the next-best thing to being there.

Other note-taking strategies

Most students take reasonably good notes but then don't use them properly. They tend to wait until just before an examination to review their notes but, by then, the notes have lost much of their meaning. Remember that active listening and note taking go hand in hand. To help you keep your notes specific, organized, and comprehensive, follow these pointers:

• Even if you disagree with a point being made by the instructor, write it down.

• Raise questions whenever appropriate.

• Develop and use a standard method of note taking, including punctuation and abbreviations.

• Keep notes in a large loose-leaf binder, which allows you to more easily use an outline form for your notes. (See *Cornell system of note taking*.) The binder also allows you to reorganize your notes easily when preparing for a test or quiz.

• Leave a few spaces blank as the lecture progresses, so additional points can be filled in later.

• Don't write down every word the lecturer says. Spend more time listening, and try to write down the main points. However, know that sometimes it's more important to write than to think.

• Listen for transition cues such as a change in vocal inflection that signify important points or a transition from one point to the next.

• Make your original notes legible enough for you to read later.

• Copy everything your instructor writes on the chalkboard. You may not be able to integrate the information with your lecture notes, but you'll have the information in your notes for referral later.

• Sit at the front of the class, where there are fewer distractions.

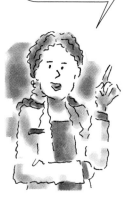

Take your notes after a film is shown in class, not during it.

Movies and other media

Taking notes from films, slides, or television differs from traditional note taking because they're associated with

Advice from the experts

Cornell system of note taking

One system of note taking called the Cornell system involves specific activities during and after a lecture. Before the lecture, obtain a large, loose-leaf binder. Use only one side of the paper. Divide your paper as shown in the illustration below.

During the lecture
Use the Notes area on the right side of the page to take notes in paragraph form. Capture general ideas, not illustrative ideas. Skip a line to show the end of an idea or thought. Use abbreviations whenever possible to save time. Write legibly.

After the lecture
Read through your notes and make them more legible as necessary. Use the Cue column to jot down ideas or key words that highlight the main aspects of the lecture. Cover the Notes area with a blank paper and describe the general ideas and concepts of the lecture using the notes in the Cue column. Use the Summary area to summarize your notes in one or two sentences.

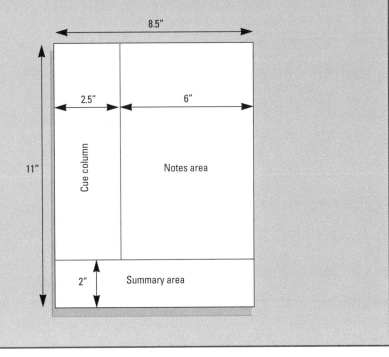

entertainment. As a result, you may not realize the importance of the information they provide. Furthermore, these types of media are usually shown in a darkened room, which is hardly conducive to note taking.

The fast pace of these formats is another stumbling block to note taking. A film or TV show doesn't provide many pauses for taking notes. For this reason, taking notes immediately after the presentation is sometimes the best alternative for recording new information. If the presentation was on film or slides, ask if you can watch the presentation again or check to see if the instructor puts the presentation on reserve in the library.

Notes on making a note-taking outline

Making a note-taking outline before the lecture gives you a basis for understanding the lecture and a chance to locate important terms, concepts, and dates beforehand. To construct a note-taking outline, divide each page of notes vertically into two sections, with one-third of the space to the left and two-thirds to the right. Then, record the chapter title and major and minor headings on the left side, estimating the amount of space that might be required for each section.

When previewing the material, survey the physical characteristics of the chapter, including length, text structure, visual aids, and term identification. Read the chapter introduction or first paragraph. Survey graphs, maps, charts, and diagrams. Look for such typographic aids as **boldface,** <u>underlining</u>, and *italics,* used to highlight important new terms or ideas. Record the terms in the outline. Finally, read the last paragraph or summary, which generally reviews the main points or conclusions of the chapter.

I'll note it myyyy way

Develop a system for taking notes that best fits your learning style and course content. Date each day's notes to serve as a reference point if you need to compare notes with someone else's or ask your instructor for clarification. If you're absent, the missing dates identify which notes you need. Other steps to personalizing your notes include:
• keeping your notes together in a notebook, preferably one with pockets that can be used to save class handouts

- bringing all necessary note-taking materials to each class
- knowing how to interpret your own shorthand
- grouping and labeling information to aid recall
- writing down facts and diagrams written on the chalkboard
- leaving room in your notes to fill in later
- skipping lines to separate important groups of ideas and writing on only one side of the paper, both of which will make it easier to read your notes later
- keeping your notes neat and your writing legible so you can read your own writing later
- organizing your notes after class
- using color coding to mark important ideas and concepts
- reading over notes as soon as possible after class, while the material is still fresh in your mind, and correcting your notes as necessary
- refraining from rewriting the text verbatim. If the instructor refers to a specific text page, go to the book and mark the information there. Remember to jot the page number in your notes and to write a brief summary later.

How much is enough?

How many notes are enough? That depends on your own confidence and your instructor's teaching style. Notes must be accurate and useful in refreshing your memory on important points.

You're probably making too few notes if you simply write down a list of facts without tying them together. Conversely, if you spend all your time writing notes, you don't have time to think about or question the material. Furthermore, you may miss an important point while writing down something less significant. Try to find a happy, effective medium.

Format tips

Be flexible enough to adapt your note-taking style to best fit the style of the instructor. One format for note taking may work well in one instructor but not another. Types of note formats that might be used include:

- *outline.* If the lecture is highly organized, an outline will probably work well. Mark main section headings with uppercase roman numerals. Mark important points under each section with capital letters and supporting points under the important points with Arabic (regular) numerals. Subordinate sets of ideas can be indented and bulleted beneath the preceding higher level.

• *thin-fat columns.* On your note paper, draw one thin column and one fat column. Use the thin column to keep track of extra notes to yourself, such as "See page 53 of text" or "Test on Tuesday." Use this column also for important facts to remember. Use the fat column to record lecture notes.

• *equal columns.* Divide your note paper into two equal columns when comparing two concepts. Put notes about one concept on one side and notes about the other on the opposite side. You'll then not only have information about both concepts but a visual way to compare and contrast the concepts.

• *idea tree.* Start with the main idea circled in the center of the writing, and then branch off facts like branches from the tree. Branch off subordinate ideas like twigs branching off of larger branches. This format is also called concept mapping.

Reviewing notes

After class, review your notes for clarity. Rewrite anything you think you might not be able to read later, particularly if you've used a number of abbreviations in your notes. Finish up open-ended notes that you didn't finish before moving on to the next topic.

Reviewing class notes can be particularly important after a disorganized lecture or one in which the instructor stated certain intentions at the beginning of the lecture but never fulfilled them. Reviewing these notes may take time and research because you may need to fill in blank spots with material from the textbook.

Reviewing your notes within 24 hours after taking them can help establish the information in your memory. If you don't look over your notes within a day, they may not make sense anymore. In addition, read your notes again before the next class to give yourself a sense of continuity.

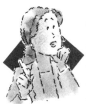

Quick quiz

1. Enumeration or sequence text is commonly preceded by such clue words as:

  A. *first, second, next,* and *then.*
  B. *primarily, mostly, hardly,* and *many.*
  C. *however, in contrast, but,* and *and yet.*

Answer: A. Enumeration or sequence text lists major points by number or in sequence and are commonly preceded by such clue words as *first, second, next,* and *then.*

2. A student is actively listening to a lecture when she:

  A. audiotapes the lecture.
  B. takes notes during the lecture.
  C. questions the accuracy of the information presented during the lecture.

Answer: B. Note taking is one of the most important parts of active listening.

3. The "S" in the LISAN method of studying stands for:

  A. signal words.
  B. staying the course.
  C. sending positive messages.

Answer: A. The letters in LISAN stands for **L**ead, **I**dea, **S**ignal words, **A**ctively listen, and **N**ote taking.

4. Listen for transition cues such as a change in vocal inflection that signify:

  A. an important point.
  B. instructor frustration.
  C. the end of the lecture.

Answer: A. Transition cues signify important points or a transition from one point to the next.

5. When your instructor shows a videotape during class, you should take notes:

  A. during class.
  B. right after class.
  C. at least 1 hour after class.

Answer: B. Because many audiovisual presentations, including videotapes, are shown in a darkened room, note taking is more difficult. Taking notes immediately after the presentation is sometimes the best alternative for recording new information.

Scoring

☆☆☆   If you answered all five questions correctly, you were really paying attention! Give yourself a free trip on the Speed Reading Railroad!

☆☆   If you answered three or four questions correctly, you must be feeling great. You've won a valuable Get the Most Out of Your Notes card!

☆   If you answered fewer than three questions correctly, not to worry. You're just a few notes away from that famed avenue of star note-takers, Chalkboardwalk!

Study strategies

Just the facts

In this chapter, you'll learn:

♦ why it's important to consider physical and environmental surroundings when preparing to study

♦ how to get started studying

♦ how the SQ4R reading-study system, the PSQ5R method of studying, reciprocal teaching, and meta-learning can help you study more effectively.

Preparing to study

Effective studying doesn't just happen. It involves carefully selecting a study site, maintaining proper lighting, settling into a comfortable position, and putting yourself into the right frame of mind.

Selecting a study area

To find the right study area, look for a distraction-free area where you can arrange your study materials properly. Make sure it has adequate lighting, is set at the right temperature, and is located among pleasant surroundings.

Distraction-free site

Before you begin to study, find a calm, comfortable place to study. As you select your study site, choose an area with the fewest distractions. (See *Distraction-free study areas*, page 130.) After you find a study site you enjoy using, keep using it for subsequent study sessions. Using the

Exercise your mind

Distraction-free study areas

Select two or three areas you think may be suitable to use as a study area. Then choose the area with the most favorable responses to these questions:

• Will I be interrupted by other people?

• Are there too many reminders of things that don't have anything to do with studying?

• Is a loud radio or television being played here?

• Does the telephone ring too often?

• Can I be here at regular intervals?

• Is the temperature comfortable or, if not, can I control the temperature?

• Can I smell cooking odors here?

same area creates familiarity and helps you begin studying as soon as you settle into the area.

Study arrangement

Next, find the arrangement for studying you most enjoy. For most students, a desk with a comfortable, straight-backed chair makes the ideal study arrangement. You can arrange your study materials on the desk and easily reach them whenever necessary. Other students feel most comfortable in a large chair or sofa, with their books and other study materials spread out on the floor at their feet.

> I find that sitting at a desk in a comfortable, straight-backed chair is best for studying.

Don't get too relaxed

You could sit cross-legged in the middle of your bed, with your study materials all around, but it's probably not a good idea. You're already familiar with your bed as a sleeping place, and you may get sleepy. Sitting under a tree with a gentle breeze blowing in a quiet place seems like a good idea, but not when the gentle breeze becomes a distraction, ruffling papers in the wind and making you constantly find your place in your notes. Choose your study arrangement carefully, weighing the value of the comfort it provides with its ability to meet your study needs.

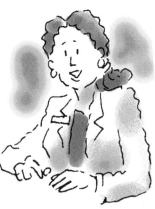

Is it just right?

To help you decide which study arrangement and study area is right for you, ask yourself these questions:
• Do I have sufficient work space?
• Can I keep the work space uncluttered?
• Do I have adequate lighting?
• Am I in a position that supports my back and eliminates muscle strain?
• Are there as few distractions as possible in the area?

Whichever study arrangement you choose, stay with it. Get into the habit of assuming your study position so you can get down to the business of studying quickly, with few distractions.

Lighting

Use either natural lighting or incandescent lighting for your study area, not fluorescent lighting. Your eyes are less likely to tire under direct light, such as from an incandescent lamp, than under indirect light.

Direct lighting is best, keeping eye fatigue at its lowest. Keep the light from shining in your eyes by using overhead light or lighting from behind. The light should shine evenly on your work.

Temperature

Choose a study area that's not too warm. Heat stress can decrease accuracy, speed, dexterity, and physical acuity. For most efficient studying, keep your study area cool — between 65° and 70° F (18° and 21° C).

Surroundings

Pleasant surroundings can greatly enhance study effectiveness. The sensations experienced while studying can be used later to trigger associations at test time. Pleasant surroundings also stimulate alertness. When creating the environment of your study site, focus on surrounding yourself with pleasant music, stimulating odors, and oxygen-providing plants.

Ahh, the pleasing sounds of Mozart...

Minimize noise distractions while you study so you won't be disturbed. Screen your telephone calls with an answering machine. Leave the television off. You might also con-

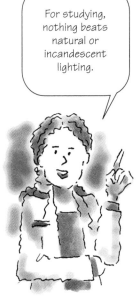

For studying, nothing beats natural or incandescent lighting.

sider adding white noise to your environment. Instrumental music, the sound of a bubbling aquarium, and muted street sounds are examples of white noise. White noise helps cover distracting background sounds, such as the sounds of traffic or your roommate talking on the phone, and fills in periods of silence. In silence, even the sound of your own tapping pencil can be annoying.

Among the forms of white noise you can use, soothing background music is preferred. Low levels of background music can promote relaxed alertness, which stimulates learning. In addition, music induces an emotional response that can be associated with a memory and improve later recall.

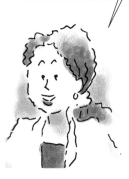

Instrumental music covers annoying noises. I generally study with Duke Ellington.

...And the odor of peppermint

The two scents that most positively stimulate attention and memory are lemon and peppermint. These scents can be found in oils, candles, room fresheners, and many other products. Other scents also exert an enhancing effect on mental alertness and relaxation. (See *Scents and the mind.*)

Gotta get some green (plants, that is)

Studying in an area where healthy plants are located can actually foster learning. Green plants remove pollutants from the air and can raise oxygen levels enough to increase productivity by as much as 10%.

Physical comfort

Your physical comfort affects your attitude about studying. When studying, make sure you assume a comfortable posture, use an appropriate reading angle, and move around periodically to enhance study effectiveness.

Sit up, like your mom used to tell you

Read while sitting in an upright position with your back straight or bent slightly forward. Other postures — particularly lying down — impair alertness and concentration.

Get the right angle

To decrease eyestrain, hold reading material at about a 45-degree angle from the flat surface of your desk or table to give you a clear view of the whole page. Reading material should also be kept at least 15″ away from your eyes.

Scents and the mind

Certain scents have been specifically identified as being influential in mental alertness and relaxation. This chart outlines those scents and how they can affect your studying.

Scent	Effect
basil	increased mental alertness
chamomile	enhanced relaxation
cinnamon	increased mental alertness
lavender	enhanced relaxation
lemon	increased mental alertness
orange	enhanced relaxation
peppermint	increased mental alertness
rose	enhanced relaxation

Get moving

Walking around periodically when studying can enhance the ability of the brain to learn new information and retain information. On average, standing increases blood flow to the brain by 5% to 15%. The greater the blood flow to the brain, the more oxygen it receives and the greater the stimulation of the neurons. So take a break about every hour to walk around, particularly if you need to ponder a point or repeat some facts to yourself. Do some stretching exercises as well to increase circulation and decrease muscle fatigue in the shoulders.

Getting started

One of the biggest challenges to effective studying is getting started. The first step in meeting that challenge is to break down large tasks into smaller ones. Several small tasks seem more achievable than one overwhelming one, and each smaller accomplishment provides moral support to finish the other tasks.

Set the compass

By taking small steps in the direction you want to go, you may end up at your destination sooner than you thought.

For instance, you may not feel like reading your assignment, but if you tell yourself that you'll read for 5 minutes, at least you'll get a little reading done. After a few minutes, tell yourself that you'll read for a few more minutes, and so on. Pretty soon, you'll have read for a half hour or maybe even an hour and be well on your way to accomplishing — if not finishing — your assignment.

Plot the course

When beginning a study session, set a course for your studying or establish a purpose for it. Ask yourself, "What do I want to get out of this session? What do I need to know from the material?" After skimming the material, decide how deeply you need to become involved with the material. You may be responsible for detailed knowledge and intricate notes or you may need only a passing acquaintance with the material. Either way, plot your course before you start.

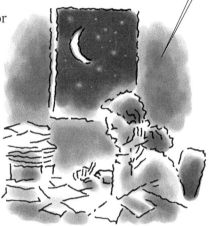

Ask yourself, "Why am I studying this? What's my goal? When can I go to bed?"

Dump those dastardly distractions

Remove the usual distractions — the telephone, television, and talk radio. Take care of your personal distractions, such as hunger or feeling hot. Schedule your study time so that it doesn't conflict with another activity you really want to do. Thinking about what you're missing can be a distraction in itself.

Find the right time to study, when you're feeling most efficient and receptive to information. Take a short break every hour to keep your study time energized. When concentration begins to lag, it's time for a break.

Special study programs

Study programs have been a popular topic since the 1940s to help students improve their studying efficiency. Four of the currently popular programs are:
- SQ4R reading-study system
- PSQ5R method
- reciprocal teaching
- metalearning.

SQ4R reading-study system

The SQ4R reading-study system involves six steps:
- *survey.* Gather information necessary to formulate study goals.
- *question.* Formulate questions to be answered.
- *read.* Seek answers for the questions you raised.
- *reflect.* Think about what the text is trying to explain or teach you.
- *recite.* Ask your original questions and recite the answer to yourself. If you can't recite the answer, read the material again. Recitation can be particularly interactive when done with another person.
- *review.* Synthesize the reading material's meaning as a whole by determining whether you answered all your original questions and met all the goals you set forth after previewing the material. Another way to review involves answering questions posed by the author at the beginning or end of the material.

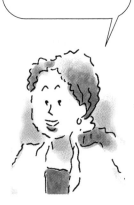

Survey, question, read, reflect, recite, review. I give it an 8. It's got a beat, but you can't dance to it.

PSQ5R method

The PSQ5R method, a system similar to the SQ4R system, involves eight steps:
- *purpose.* Determine your purpose for reading.
- *survey.* Preview the material quickly.
- *question.* Raise questions you think the reading should answer.
- *read selectively.* Read with your purpose and questions in mind.
- *recite.* Mentally repeat what you've learned as you go along.
- *reduce-record.* Write what you've learned in outline — or reduced — form.
- *reflect.* Mentally elaborate on what you've learned, comparing the material to previously learned material, categorizing it, or otherwise reorganizing the material.
- *review.* Survey your "reduced" notes (the outline) within 24 hours to enhance your knowledge of the material.

Reciprocal teaching

In reciprocal teaching, the student is taught to:
• summarize the content of a passage
• ask a question about the central point
• clarify the difficult parts of the material
• predict what will come next.

> Reciprocal teaching makes the student be the teacher.

Steps involved

Reciprocal teaching starts when you and the instructor silently read a short passage in a book or journal. Then the instructor provides a model by summarizing, questioning, clarifying, and predicting based on the reading. You'll then read another passage, but this time you'll assume the instructor's role by summarizing, questioning, clarifying, and predicting. The instructor may prompt you by giving clues, guidance, and encouragement to help you master these strategies.

Easy on the shift

To make reciprocal teaching effective, the shift from the instructor having control of the teaching process to you having the control must be gradual. Furthermore, the instructor must match the difficulty of the task to your own particular abilities.

Metalearning

Metalearning is a method of learning that involves asking yourself a series of questions:
• Why am I reading or listening to this?
• What's the overall content?
• What are the orientation questions?
• What's important here?
• Can I paraphrase or summarize the information?
• How can I organize the information?
• How can I draw the information?
• Can I associate the information?
• How does the information fit what I know?

Why am I reading or listening to this?

In the metalearning process, state your purpose briefly. Your purpose and goals set the stage for your study session. In the case of a lecture, ask yourself what you want to get out of the class. Try to anticipate what's coming next.

What's the overall content?

Preview the material before reading or attending the lecture. For long or complicated material, translate your preview into a chapter map or outline. You might also want to write what you know about the topic and what you'd like to know or expect to learn about it. This type of warm-up starts the process of generating questions, makes you aware of what you don't know about a topic, puts you on the lookout for answers to questions, and provides a resource on which to draw later. After previewing the material, summarize the chapter in a few sentences and outline brief answers to whatever review questions might be included in the book.

What are the orientation questions?

Be on the lookout for orientation questions, which commonly appear on tests. An orientation question provides background information about a topic or concept and can take a number of forms, including those that ask about definitions, examples, types, relationships, or comparisons.

The purpose for identifying orientation questions is to see how many questions you can ask about the material and how many different answers you can create for each. Don't be afraid to guess at the answer. Later, when you find out the actual answer, compare it with the one you gave. If you don't find the answer to your question, try looking in a different source.

What's important here?

Identify which information you should focus on, skim, or ignore. If you can't decide whether something is important, assume it is. Pay attention to your initial responses to the material. If something surprises or confuses you, there may be a gap in your understanding of the information.

Each subject contains important terms you should know. Textbooks typically call your attention to them with italic or bold print or include the term in a glossary. Isolated facts or other details may be important — or not — depending on your purpose for studying.

Can I paraphrase or summarize the information?

Paraphrasing a concept — putting it into your own words — can help you better understand the concept and immediately identify gaps in your learning. If you can't paraphrase a concept, you probably don't understand it well. To paraphrase effectively, use your own words and as few words as possible.

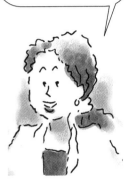

Let's see how many questions I can ask about the material. Questioning will help me learn.

How can I organize the information?

Organizing information allows your brain to place pieces of information into groups or categories so you can see patterns, connections, and relationships. Try to keep the number of groups manageable — fewer than 10 — so the information doesn't become too complicated to remember.

For example, if you need to learn the differences among several drugs, you might create categories that group the drugs by indications or adverse reactions only. That way, you can study the drugs in groups according to something they have in common, rather than studying them separately.

You might also consider organizing the information visually by using a mind-mapping technique. By writing the associations you're making among pieces of information, you're making a record of your natural thought processes about the information and will be more prepared to recall it later.

How can I draw the information?

Representing information as pictures can be a great help in building understanding. Draw a picture of the information. The process of drawing the information can improve your understanding of the information and help move the information into your long-term memory.

Can I associate the information?

Associating new information with a song, rhyme, odor, or other environmental trigger can ease later recall. Use association and other memory-enhancing techniques to improve retention and recall.

How does the information fit with what I know?

Your accumulated knowledge and understanding of the material helps you decide what's important and condense new information into easier-to-manage pieces. If you already have a solid foundation of knowledge about the topic, you can more easily learn new aspects of the topic.

Other ways to engage the brain

Raising other questions can also help engage your brain and enhance retention and later recall. Some of these questions include:

- How is this information significant?
- What does it tell us about other things?
- Is this a fact or someone's opinion?
- How can this be verified?
- Does it depend on a particular point of view?
- What if...?
- Where have I seen something like this before?
- What does that suggest about this?
- What does this remind me of?

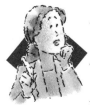

Quick quiz

1. For most efficient studying, keep the temperature in your study area between:

    A. 60° and 65° F (16° and 18° C).
    B. 65° and 70° F (18° and 21° C).
    C. 70° and 75° F (21° and 24° C).

Answer: B. For most efficient studying, keep your study area cool — between 65° and 70° F (18° and 21° C).

2. The two scents that most positively stimulate attention and memory are:

    A. lemon and oregano.
    B. parsley and peppermint.
    C. lemon and peppermint.

Answer: C. The two scents that most positively stimulate attention and memory are lemon and peppermint.

3. The four Rs in the SQ4R reading-study system are:

    A. read, respond, recite, and reflect.
    B. read, 'rite, reflect, and review.
    C. read, reflect, recite, and review.

Answer: C. The SQ4R reading-study system involves six steps: survey, question, read, reflect, recite, and review.

Scoring

☆☆☆   If you answered all three questions correctly, wow! You've won first prize at the Metalearning Center Festival. Congrats!

☆☆   If you answered two questions correctly, pat yourself on the back! You're our favorite reciprocal instructor!

☆   If you answered fewer than two questions correctly, not to worry. You'll be mastering the SQ4R — and maybe even the vaulted PSQ5R — study strategy in no time!

Test-taking strategies

Just the facts

In this chapter, you'll learn:

♦ how to prepare mentally for a test, including how to construct a study plan, relax, and develop a positive attitude

♦ how to prepare physically for a test

♦ how objective examinations focus on recalling specific information

♦ how subjective examinations focus on your ability to explain ideas

♦ how learning about the results of a test can help you prepare for future tests.

Preparing for the test

Being a top test taker demands preparation. The first step in that preparation is to recognize elements of test anxiety that may be preventing you from reaching your best performance. After you've identified test anxiety elements, you can prepare your mind and body for the test.

Recognize test anxiety

Test anxiety comes in many forms and may occur before the test or during the test itself. Types of test anxiety include:

• freezing up, in which your brain doesn't register the meaning of questions or you have to read test questions several times to comprehend them

• panicking about a difficult question or the thought of time running out
• worrying about the test
• being easily distracted, spending time daydreaming about ways to escape rather than completing the test itself
• feeling nervous, which can prevent you from putting in the time necessary to succeed
• physical symptoms such as nausea, muscle tension, headache, and sweating
• feeling a lack of interest in the test or topic. Some students find it easier not to care than to face their anxiety about performing well.

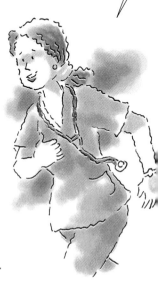

A little anxiety can help me focus better on the crisis at hand.

A little anxiety is OK

Feeling slightly anxious — but not *too* anxious — can improve your mental clarity and provide greater focus. Complacency, on the other hand, is more likely to result in falling short of your goals. If you find that you're consistently underperforming or feeling the physical effects of test anxiety — such as exhaustion, vague discomfort, and an inability to remember information — test anxiety may be getting the best of you.

Prepare the mind

Most successful students use a combination of techniques to prepare themselves mentally to perform well on tests. To cope with test anxiety, study well, relax, stay positive, and take well-planned breaks.

Studying well is the best reward

Studying well can be the best antidote for test anxiety. The feeling of accomplishment that comes with an effective study regimen can banish many of the fears that cause test anxiety.

Relaxation modification

Relaxation and other stress-reduction techniques can reduce test anxiety and give you the clarity of mind necessary to study effectively. Rhythmic breathing and meditation are two of the many techniques you might consider to reduce test anxiety.

Accentuate the positive

Test anxiety commonly stems from low self-esteem. Make an effort to think positively about the test experience. Tell yourself, "I can do it!" You'll be amazed how often positive results follow positive thinking.

Take a break

Mild, short-term test anxiety can often be reduced by taking a short break. If you feel anxious during a test, sharpen your pencil or get a drink of water. If you feel anxious while studying, give yourself a quick break away from studying. Sometimes anxiety is your body's way of saying, "I need a few minutes off."

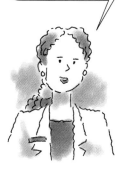

Telling yourself, "I can do it!" can help combat test anxiety.

Prepare the body

Many students, even those with rigorous study habits, neglect their bodies when preparing for a test. Maximum test performance depends on meeting the need for proper rest, nutrition, and overall health. Physical preparedness is basic to improving your test-taking skills.

R and R

Rest and relaxation can overcome fatigue following intense mental or physical exertion. You can accomplish more when you feel rested and relaxed than when you're fatigued. To make sure you get enough rest and relaxation:
- get a sufficient amount of sleep
- change activities periodically
- exercise regularly
- relax periodically by watching television, listening to music, talking to friends, or reading a book.

Sit straight

Your posture during studying and examinations can affect your mood. Slouching not only hurts your back but can also make you feel sluggish and disinterested. Maintain good posture, and watch your focus improve.

Eat nutritious test treats

Because nutrition affects your physical well-being, it also affects your study habits and test-taking skills. Because class time, work time, and study time may conflict with eating on a regular schedule, counterbalance odd mealtimes with nutritious snacks or meals.

When you're sick

Eat nutritiously to sharpen your test-taking skills.

Even when you're in strong physical condition, you may become too ill to study properly to take a test. Don't neglect symptoms of illness in favor of studying for an upcoming test; you'll most likely feel ill during the test and, as a result, perform poorly. If you become ill, contact the instructor as soon as possible. This communicates your concern about missing the test and helps alleviate your own anxiety about missing it. Follow all of your doctor's guidelines for getting well again, including taking medications as prescribed and resting as much as the doctor advises.

Stay in the habit

When a test is coming up, don't do anything that will upset your sense of normalcy. If you normally walk 30 minutes a day after lunch, don't jog during that time to relieve stress. You'll probably end up being sore, tired, *and* stressed. If you normally sleep 8 hours a night, avoid pulling an all-nighter. You may end up throwing off your sleep pattern and becoming sleep-deprived — not a healthy state for your brain just before a test.

Planning for the test

Successful students think about upcoming tests long before the day of the examination. They learn all they can about the test itself and then construct their study time accordingly.

Learn about the test

Before studying for a test, know what kind of test it's going to be. If you know what kind of test to expect, your study time will be more focused. For objective tests (short-answer, sentence-completion, multiple-choice, matching, and true-false), focus your study on knowing facts and details and being able to recognize related material. For essay or oral tests, preparation includes being able to argue persuasively about several general topics and to back up those arguments with details.

In any case, you'll need to find out key pieces of information about the test to prepare properly, including facts about the test format and objectives, availability of past tests, and the overall structure of the class.

Size it up

To find out about a test, ask the instructor. Many instructors explain the format of their tests to the whole class. Others inform only those students who ask. For those instructors especially, be sure to ask about test format. When faced with an upcoming test, ask:
• Will the test be comprehensive or cover certain chapters only?
• How many questions will it contain?
• How will the questions be weighted?
• Will it be subjective or objective?
• Will it require that I apply knowledge or just know facts?
• How important is this test to my final grade?
• What can I bring to the test? Will calculators be allowed? Will formulas be supplied?
• Who is making the test?
• Who will grade the test?
• Will it be a special type of examination, such as a take-home test or an open-book test?

Look to the past

If you've already taken tests in this course, you may already have an idea of what the upcoming test will be like. Past experience may tell you that the previous test focused on details rather than principles or that it contained an occasional "trick" question. If this is your first test in the course, check for copies of past examinations. These may be available from the instructor or be on file with the instructor's department or college library. Study the examinations for ideas about what to expect, but don't expect the exact same questions or directions.

Sometimes old tests are on file at the library.

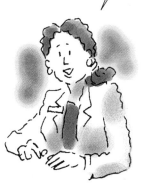

Look to the class

The structure of the class can also yield clues about an upcoming test. Which topics have been singled out for greater emphasis or more detailed explanation? Does the instructor emphasize details or global ideas? Some instructors give optional review sessions before an examination. In such a case, attend the session and be prepared. Write down questions you want to ask before the examination.

Create a study plan

Get started early when studying for an upcoming test. Most instructors explain at the beginning of the semester when tests will be administered. Note test dates in your semester calendar. If the dates haven't been announced, ask the instructor for approximate dates of the examinations.

Plan ahead

Make an organized, continuous study plan. Studying every day for the week before a test keeps the material fresh and clear in your mind. Plan enough time to review lecture notes several times and to rehearse the information.

Give yourself at least a week to study for an examination. Reviewing your notes after each class is recommended practice for helping you to understand and keep up with the material but, when preparing for a test, more intense review is needed. Sometimes the instructor gives an unannounced in-class quiz. In case of a "pop" quiz, you'll be glad you reviewed material covered in each class.

Each day, plan how much time you'll devote to studying, what time of day you'll study, and where you'll study. If you plan to study with a partner, set up the meeting times early.

Use a calendar to construct your study plan. Mark what you'll study each day and for how long.

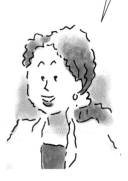

Assemble your sources

Gather review materials together. Compile information about the main terms, facts, concepts, themes, problems, questions, and issues stressed in the lectures. The most likely sources for this information include course notes and the textbook.

The textbook's index and glossary are valuable resources for finding important topics and definitions of key terms. Supplementary reading and handouts supplied by the instructor should also be available for review. Keep in mind that material assigned by the instructor but not discussed in class may appear on the test — not just information covered in class.

Read and review

When you begin reviewing your class notes in preparation for an examination, be sure to go over your notes and reading materials more than once. Don't expect to remember everything about a topic in one reading.

The first pass at the material serves to refresh the information and lay a foundation for subsequent passes. Each review becomes easier than the last because the information is fresh and you can anticipate the next topic or sequence of ideas. Take a break between review sessions to let your brain ponder relationships within the material.

Make your own cheat sheets

Condense your notes to a one-page summary sheet. Then reconstruct the notes from memory, picturing the placement of notes on the page. Gain command of the material by reciting details. Review techniques for various types of tests include:

• For mathematical or scientific testing, drill yourself by rewriting equations and graphs. Practice writing mathematical symbols so that you can reproduce them easily. Practice solving sample problems. If you have particular trouble with certain mathematical expressions or graphs, write them out separately and keep them with you to look at from time to time.

• For short-answer tests, make a list of important terms and write the definition of each. Think of an example for each term.

• For essay questions, look at old essay assignments and examinations. Choose a topic that relates to what you've been learning in class. Write an outline and thesis statement, then flesh out the essay, giving yourself as much time as you'd have for a real examination.

Here I am on Saturday again, taking a practice test in the classroom. What we do to succeed, eh?

Dress rehearsal

For every test, try to compile a simulated test based on material from your instructor or review questions in your text. Administer the test under testlike conditions, preferably in the same room where you'll take the real examination and for the same length of time. This dress rehearsal will familiarize you with the testing conditions and may alleviate some of the anxiety about facing an unfamiliar situation.

Test day

On the day of the test, you can take several actions to make sure you do your best on the examination, including:

- resting
- eating small meals
- avoiding caffeinated drinks and foods
- exercising briefly
- having your test materials ready to go
- arriving to class on time, without rushing
- reading the test directions
- budgeting test time efficiently.

Take care of your body

You should get at least 6 hours of sleep the night before a test. In addition, try to wake up at your regular time and eat a normal breakfast without breaking routine. Don't overeat; doing so will cause your body to work harder on digesting the meal than in coming up with answers for the test.

Be careful as well not to overstimulate yourself with caffeinated drinks and foods. Caffeine-related stimulation can distract you and make you jittery for the test.

Brief exercise before a test can invigorate your mind by increasing cerebral circulation. Be careful not to exercise too much, though; exercise just enough to get your blood moving.

Take one last, leisurely look

Review your summary sheet casually. If you have last-minute facts or formulas to remember, commit them to memory as close to examination time as possible. This information will most likely be stored in short-term memory and won't last long. Jot these facts down as soon as the test begins.

Prepare your supplies

Gather all the supplies you'll need for the examination, especially a watch and extra pens. During a timed test, you may worry excessively if you don't know how long you've been working and how much time is left. Bring pens, pen-

> A short, leisurely jog is just what I need to wake up my mind before a test.

cils, erasers, paper, a calculator, and other items as needed and allowed.

Dress comfortably in layers. If the room is hot, peel off a layer. If it's cold, add a sweater. Bring an easy-to-eat snack and water if you think you may become distracted by hunger or thirst. Be sure to prepare these supplies well in advance of the test so you're not rushing around immediately before you head to class. In fact, you might consider keeping these items in a test kit, which you can grab before each test and restock afterward. The night before a test, put the test kit with your car keys or other item you *know* you'll be taking to the test, so you won't forget it.

Be the early bird

Be 5 to 10 minutes early for your test. Select the seat you want, preferably one with the least potential for distractions. If the room is poorly lit, sit beneath a light fixture. Stay away from seats near the door. If you still have time, continue reviewing your condensed notes. Avoid listening to other students chat among themselves, especially if they're discussing the examination. Their conversation may make you unduly anxious and cause you to concern yourself needlessly with material you already know well.

Let the instructions instruct

When you take your first look at the test, don't let your eye jump to the first question. Instead, read the directions and listen carefully to verbal instructions. Underline, circle, or otherwise mark important instructions, such as "fill in the circles," "copy the question," or "show your work." Look at the sample questions if there are any, and work them through.

Next, skim through the test for an overall sense of the questions and their level of difficulty. Read the questions that require lengthy writing. By reviewing the questions in advance, your brain can work on answers to longer questions while you're addressing shorter questions.

In essay questions, underline key words and jot down notes that you don't want to forget when you come back to answer the question completely. For example, you may want to write dates or points you want to make about a question you plan on answering last.

> Even if you're anxious to start the test, it's important to read the directions first.

Budget your time

After reading the directions and previewing the test, determine a budget for your test time. Take into consideration:
• how much time you've been given to complete the examination
• the total number of questions
• the type and difficulty of each question
• the point value for each question.

If you have a choice of questions, decide which ones you intend to answer and in which order you plan to answer them. If, during the test, you start to lag behind the schedule you set, be flexible. Rebound by deciding how you can best use your remaining time.

Test types

You may be faced with any combination of a variety of types of tests, each of which requires its own strategies. Types of tests include objective tests, such as multiple-choice and true-false tests, subjective tests such as essays, and other types of tests, such as vocabulary, reading comprehension, open-book, take-home, oral, and standardized tests.

Objective

In an objective test, only one correct answer to a question is possible. These tests primarily measure your ability to recall information. Objective questions are frequently used in standardized examinations. Types of objective tests include:
• multiple-choice
• true-false
• short-answer
• sentence-completion
• problem-solving.

First things first

For all objective tests, first look over the entire test to determine the number of questions in the test. Try to answer the questions in the order they appear. Mark difficult questions, and then move on. You can return to difficult questions after you've reached the end of the test and have time left. You may be more able to handle these questions because your brain has had a chance to think about them. In addition, other questions may prompt you to remember the correct answer.

Multiple-choice

Observe these principles when taking a multiple-choice examination:

• Read the question carefully. Qualifying phrases such as *except* and *all of the following* provide important clues to the correct answer.

• Think of an answer before looking at the options. Then try to match your answer to one of the options. Even if you find a match right away, read all the answers anyway. You may find that another option comes closer to the answer you originally supplied.

• Use the process of elimination to narrow your choices. Eliminating clearly wrong options greatly improves your odds of selecting the correct option.

• Work quickly. Read each question through, answer it, and move on to the next question.

Selecting the "best"

Sometimes, test instructions say to select the "best" answer. In such a case, there may be more than one right answer, but one may be better or more appropriate than the others. In these cases, prioritize to determine which answer best responds to the question.

When prioritizing, think of well-known principles or theories. For a question that asks what you would do first, for instance, think of Maslow's hierarchy of needs. Physical needs are always more important than psychological needs, so meeting nutritional demands is automatically more important than establishing a trusting relationship.

In a well-constructed test, all options are plausible. Therefore, go back to the question and look for a clue word that makes one answer better than the others. Some test makers deliberately put a plausible — but incorrect — answer first. To avoid picking the first answer that appears, read all answers before deciding which is correct.

Some tests offer more than one correct response. Read all of the responses and choose the best answer.

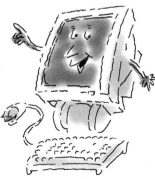

When it just seems right

Sometimes, questions and correct responses are taken right out of textbook or lecture notes. So if you recognize particular words or phrases in one of the options or the question and one option seems like the right combination, choose that option; it's probably right.

Be alert for "attractive distracters," words that *look like* the word to be defined but aren't. For example, if *illusion* is the correct answer, *allusion* might be used as a decoy among the answers.

Use your time wisely

When you've finished the test, go back and read the directions again to make sure you've followed them. Check that you've answered the questions in the areas where they were supposed to be answered. Check the questions you flagged for further review. Finally, review all questions if you have time. Change answers only if you're convinced they need to be changed to be correct. Trust your first impressions; they're usually accurate.

True-false

In general, true-false questions assess your recognition of information rather than your ability to recall it and concentrate on simple facts and details. Most true-false statements are straightforward and based on key words or phrases from the textbook or lectures. Always decide whether the statement is completely true before you mark it true. If only part of it is true, then the whole statement is false.

Take the hint

One word can turn an otherwise true statement into a false one or a false one into a true one. Pay special attention to:
- all
- always
- because
- generally
- never
- none
- only
- sometimes
- usually.

> Pay attention to small words, such as "always" and "never." They're vital for selecting the correct response.

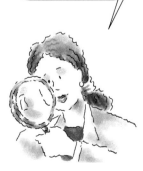

Short-answer and sentence-completion

Short-answer test items usually consist of one or two specific sentences, such as writing a definition or giving a formula. Sentence-completion items typically consist of a single sentence in which you're asked to fill in a specific word or phrase.

Plan of attack

To take a short-answer or sentence-completion test, break the items into three categories according to the items you:

☝ know without hesitation

✌ should be able to answer if you think for a minute

🖐 have no idea about.

Answer the questions you know first. Then attack the questions that need more thought. Finally, answer all remaining questions.

Don't blank out on blanks

Sentence-completion, or fill-in-the-blank, questions generally ask for an exact wording from memory. Use the length and number of blanks provided as a clue to the correct answer. Make sure the grammar is consistent. When in doubt, guess; even if you make a generalized guess, you may receive partial credit. Many times, the question itself will contain a clue to the correct answer. For example, a date may help you narrow the scope of answers simply by providing a point of historical reference.

Look at the number and length of blanks in the question. Is there more than one blank? Are the blanks long or short? Many instructors deliberately indicate when they expect one word, two words, or three by using that number of blanks. The instructor may also use long blanks for long answers and short blanks for short answers.

Problem-solving examinations

Tests that require problem-solving skills are used mainly in quantitative subjects, such as math and science. To approach a problem-solving examination, first read through all of the problems before answering any. Underline key words in the directions and important data in the problem. Jot down thoughts that come to mind, such as specific formulas or possible approaches for solving the problem.

Then move to the next question, and repeat the same pro-
cedure.

Easy ones first

Work on the easiest problems first; return to the more difficult ones later. Working on simple problems first will
help build your confidence and warm up your brain for
the more difficult problems to come.

Put it all on the page

Show all of your work. If you make a mistake, the
instructor can see where you went wrong and at
least give you partial credit. Be careful and deliberate about your calculations so you don't make
computational errors. Check that your answer
meets all of the requirements of the problem. In
addition, check that your answers make sense. If
your answer indicates that you would give a patient
20 pills, does that make sense? If not, check your
work again.

Try a different approach

If you have trouble solving a problem, approach it in a different manner. Think about similar problems from class or
homework and the methods used to solve them. These
are typically the methods used in the test except that the
ones in the test use different numbers or scenarios. Keep
in mind that there's usually more than one way to solve a
problem. If one method doesn't work, try another.

> Show all your
> calculations. Even
> if the answer isn't
> correct, you may
> get partial credit.

Subjective tests

In a subjective test, such as an essay test, no single correct answer exists. Instead, a person grading the test
judges how well each essay demonstrates understanding
of the material. Follow these steps for successfully completing an essay test:
• Read all directions, underlining important words and
phrases.
• Read all questions even if you need to answer only three
of them. Jot down facts and thoughts about each topic.
• Mark the time you estimate it will take to complete each
question.
• Outline your answer.
• Write the answer.

• Read the directions and question again. Review your answer. Proofread, and make corrections.

Know what to do

Read all directions first. Failure to do so can result in points being taken off. For instance, the directions may say to supply three supporting facts for each point of view. If you provide only one or two facts, you may lose points.

When reading the directions for the first time, underline key points so you can refer to them quickly as you write. Unless the directions say otherwise, double-space your essay and write only on the right-hand pages of the test booklet. Both techniques provide room for information to be added and for comments from the instructor.

Know what to choose

After reading all directions, read all questions, quickly jotting down what you know about each topic, including facts, formulas, names, dates, ideas, and impressions. Later, when you write your outline, you'll have facts and figures handy to plug into the essay quickly. In addition, if you have a choice of questions for the test, you'll know which topics you know the most about by looking at how many notes you've written for each.

> If the essay question is worth half the test grade, plan to spend half your time on it.

Know how long it will take

If a single essay question is worth, say, 50% of your grade, plan to spend 50% of your time on that question. Break this time allotment down further to include the time required to organize an outline, write the essay, and check your work.

Know how to organize your material

When creating an outline, first write your thesis statement to guide you in writing the rest of the essay. Choose a title, even if one isn't required. The title, like the thesis, also helps guide the direction of your arguments.

When organizing your outline, use the five-paragraph format as a guide. (See *Five-paragraph format*, page 156.) Content and organization typically account for most of your test grade. If you run out of time while writing an essay, you may be able to submit your outline, which shows your organization and intent.

Advice from the experts

Five-paragraph format

The five-paragraph format is an easy-to-follow structure for answering an essay question that asks you to state and support an opinion. Use it to get yourself started, especially when pressed for time.

Paragraph	Content
1	Introduction, in which you briefly outline the direction your argument will take and list the three main points you'll illustrate
2	First point, including at least two supporting facts
3	Second point, including at least two supporting facts
4	Third point, including at least two supporting facts
5	Conclusion, which pulls together the three main points into one final summary statement

Know what to write

Follow your outline when you write, and get to the point quickly. Your thesis statement should restate the question or answer the question succinctly. Use the introduction to tell the instructor what you're going to say. If the question says to "explain" or "summarize," for example, be sure to do just that.

Guided by your outline, make your points and supporting statements in the body of the essay. Each paragraph should have a topic statement, which, in turn, should be relevant to your thesis statement. Incorporate the facts and thoughts you jotted down at the beginning of the test. Write simple, direct, specific sentences that follow each other logically.

The conclusion should restate your thesis, drawing together the points made in the body of the essay. The conclusion tells the instructor that you had a point to make and you made it.

Know what to review

When you've finished writing your essay, go back and read the question and directions again. (See *Essay checklist.*) Make sure you've answered the question and that

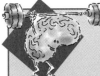

Exercise your mind

Essay checklist

After completing an essay question, check your work. Ask yourself these questions to determine whether you've covered all the points you intended to cover.

Content

- Did you stick to your original point of view?
- Have you proven each argument?
- Have you provided examples?
- Have you clearly distinguished facts from opinions?
- Have you mentioned exceptions to your general statements?

Organization

- Did you open with a topic sentence?
- Does the topic sentence address the question?
- Did you follow your outline?
- Did you cover all the points in your original outline?
- Does your ending pull together all points without adding new information?

Writing mechanics

- Does every sentence say what you intended it to say?
- Are you sure of the meanings of all the words?
- Are spelling, grammar, punctuation, and sentence structure correct?
- Is your work neat and your handwriting legible?

you've addressed all the points in the directions. Then read your essay slowly and carefully, proofreading for grammatical errors and legibility. (See *Writing mechanics for essay questions,* page 158.) Make corrections where necessary.

Other types

Other types of tests include:
- vocabulary
- reading comprehension
- open-book and take-home

Advice from the experts

Writing mechanics for essay questions

Answering an essay question involves providing the correct information, of course, but it also involves presenting the information in a readable format. Like a finely tuned car, a finely crafted essay shows that the author pays attention to mechanical details. Following certain tips for mechanically precise writing will help you write clear, compelling answers to essay questions.

Punctuation and word choice

• Avoid semicolons, exclamation marks, and parenthetical statements. Many inexperienced writers use semicolons incorrectly and exclamation marks too frequently. Parenthetical statements can knock a sentence off track.

• Avoid using a big word when a smaller one will do. Using unnecessarily long words or jargon can confuse your reader and detract from the clarity of your response. Keep it simple, and your instructor will be able to judge your knowledge more clearly.

• Avoid fragments and run-ons. A fragment is an incomplete sentence, such as *Because the laboratory technologist is responsible for monitoring blood bank supplies.* A run-on is a long sentence typically formed by joining two or three other sentences without using proper punctuation or linking words.

• Avoid slang, nonstandard language, or profanity. Keep your tone professional throughout.

Content and transitions

• Support all opinions with facts or other supporting information.

• Use transitions properly to give your writing a smooth flow. For example, if you introduce a term or concept at the end of one paragraph, use the term or refer to the concept in the first sentence of the next paragraph.

• When working on lined paper, skip every other line as you write. Skipping lines makes it easier for the instructor to read your response and also allows for extra room in which to write additional information later.

• oral
• standardized.

Vocabulary tests

A vocabulary test assesses your ability to remember the meaning of a word or use it correctly. Vocabulary tests are often used when studying foreign languages or in fields that employ specialized terminology.

Winning with word tests

The following strategies are useful when you're faced with a vocabulary test:

• Avoid decoy options that look like the correct answer but aren't.

• Choose grammatically correct answers only.

• If you don't know the meaning of a word, try to remember where you've heard it and how it was used in a sentence. Select the answer that seems closest in meaning.

• Try to determine what part of speech the word is — for example, is it a noun or verb? Knowing a word's part of speech helps put the word into grammatical context and give you a clue about the meaning.

• Apply your knowledge of other languages. If you studied Latin, for instance, you may be able to derive the correct answer by looking at the unknown word's root. Look also at the word's prefix or suffix for clues.

Reading comprehension tests

In a reading comprehension test, you'll be asked to read a particular passage and then answer questions based on the passage. For these tests, read the *questions* first and then the passage. That way, you can focus on finding answers to the questions as you read.

Just the facts

After you read the passage, base your answers entirely on facts given in the passage. Applying outside knowledge can cost you points. Check your answers to make sure you've completely answered the questions.

Open-book and take-home

In an open-book or take-home examination, you're allowed to refer to your textbooks or notes. These tests de-emphasize memorization and encourage critical thinking. They're often graded more strictly than other tests based on your ability to eliminate factual errors. Neatness and grammar may count more heavily because you're given time to find and correct those errors.

Know your textbook

Strategies for taking an open-book or take-home examination include:

> If you glance at the questions first in a reading comprehension test, then you can look for answers while you read the passage.

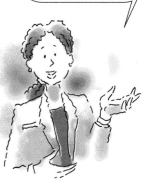

- Use the index and table of contents extensively.
- Don't copy your essays from the book. Use as many sources and resources as you're allowed. Treat the assignment like writing a paper.
- For some open-book tests, the instructor may allow students to bring only one page of notes. In such a case, organize and condense as much information as possible onto that one paper.
- Check your answers. Make sure you answered the questions without adding new, unsupported thoughts at the end.
- Proofread your work.

Oral tests

In an oral examination, you need to speak clearly, fluently, and without much time to prepare an answer. If you're allowed to choose a topic in advance, prepare as completely as if you were writing an essay. Choose a limited topic on which you can remain focused and give many supporting details. Try to make at least three points during the examination and support each point with three pieces of evidence.

Say it again, Sam

Practice for an oral test the same way you would prepare for a written test. Rehearse your answers in a simulated testing situation. Practice public speaking so you feel comfortable speaking in front of an audience. To help you get through your oral test:

- Dress appropriately, and look neat. Your physical appearance can make a positive or negative impression on your audience.
- Maintain control of your voice. Speak clearly and in measured tones. Avoid speaking quickly, mumbling, or letting your voice become too excited and "squeaky."
- Look at your audience. If you can't look directly at someone in the audience, look at a reference point in the audience. Looking at a reference point in the audience gives audience members the impression that you're looking at them. You might also look just above the heads of the people in the audience.
- If the oral test involves giving a speech, prepare notes and do most of your speaking without reading. If you read directly from your notes, you might sound ill-prepared.

Oh, yeah. I luuuuv open-book tests. Can't you tell? Help!

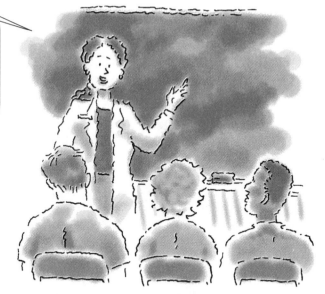

Practice will help me speak clearly and fluently during my oral examination.

• Use language you're comfortable with. Don't use offensive language or words you don't know how to pronounce. In preparing, practice pronouncing the names of people or places that may come up during your test.
• Treat questions seriously. If you're allowed to take notes, write down questions asked of you. This is particularly helpful if the question contains several parts. If you don't understand what the questioner is asking, request a clarification. Always repeat or rephrase the question yourself so you're sure you understand it.
• Unless you know how to answer a question immediately, take a moment to organize your thoughts after being asked a question.
• If you don't know the answer to a question, explain why. Perhaps the answer falls outside your realm of expertise.
• Exit gracefully. When your test is over, collect yourself and your papers, and thank the audience members for their attention.

Standardized tests

Standardized tests — for example, the Graduate Record Examination (GRE), Millers Analogy Test (MAT), and Scholastic Aptitude Test (SAT) — are used for placement and admissions purposes. The test scores for standardized tests become a permanent part of your academic record.

Exercise your mind

Test review checklist

Reviewing your test after it has been corrected can help clarify where you went wrong and what areas you need to concentrate on for the next test. When your test is handed back, ask yourself these questions:

• What was your biggest problem overall?

• In general, what types of comments did the instructor make?

• Did you prepare for this test properly?

• Did you make careless errors? If so, how can you avoid doing the same in the future?

• What else can you learn from your mistakes?

Always prepare before taking a standardized test by practicing under simulated test conditions. Use materials prepared by the same people who publish the actual test or materials designed specifically to replicate the actual test.

Numerous practice books and software are available for nearly every major standardized test. Take advantage of these books, using their self-tests to practice under simulated test conditions. Practice questions may also be available on the Internet, depending on the test.

Test review

Tests provide you and your instructor with valuable information to evaluate your performance and judge your progress. Most instructors review the tests with the class after the examination. Review your examination when it's returned to you. (See *Test review checklist.*) Reflect carefully on instructor comments on the test, especially comments on an essay test. They can tell you not only about mistakes you've made but also how you can better fulfill that particular instructor's expectations.

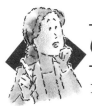

Quick quiz

1. Physical effects of test anxiety include:
- A. dizziness.
- B. exhaustion.
- C. numbness or tingling in the hands.

Answer: B. If you find that you're consistently feeling the physical effects of test anxiety — such as exhaustion, vague discomfort, and an inability to remember information — test anxiety may be getting the best of you.

2. Types of objective tests include:
- A. multiple-choice and essay.
- B. essay and short-answer.
- C. short-answer and multiple-choice.

Answer: C. Objective tests include short-answer, sentence-completion, multiple-choice, matching, and true-false.

3. In a reading comprehension test, you should *first* read the:
- A. grading criteria.
- B. passage.
- C. questions.

Answer: C. In a reading comprehension test, you'll be asked to read a passage and then answer questions based on the passage. For these tests, however, read the *questions* first and then the passage.

4. The purpose of using standardized tests is:
- A. midterm evaluation.
- B. instructor evaluation.
- C. placement and admission.

Answer: C. Standardized tests — for example, the Graduate Record Examination (GRE), Millers Analogy Test (MAT), and Scholastic Aptitude Test (SAT) — are used for placement and admissions purposes.

Scoring

☆☆☆   If you answered all four questions correctly, you make the grade! Not only have you aced this test but you've earned the coveted Premier Test Taker of the Year award. Congrats!

☆☆   If you answered three questions correctly, way to go! You've earned the esteemed Essayist of the Month award. Super!

☆   If you answered fewer than three questions correctly, you're probably just test-anxious. Not to worry, you're next in line to receive the multifaceted Multiple-Choice Master award. Gadzooks!

Overcoming obstacles

No matter how well you prepare for class, how much you study, how intent you are on your goal, you'll face obstacles along your journey through school. Things may happen that you're unprepared for or don't know how to handle. This special section anticipates those obstacles and answers your questions about handling them.

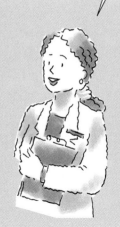

Never put off until tomorrow what you should at least start today.

I'm a procrastinator. How can I avoid getting behind in my studies because I procrastinate?

Procrastination is one of the most common obstacles faced by students trying to get ready for a test or homework assignment. When you procrastinate, you use your time inefficiently and risk not reaching the goals you've set for yourself.

When time is used inefficiently, many things scheduled to get done don't get done. If you're having trouble using your time efficiently, use these principles of time management:

• Keep track of how much time you spend on each assignment. Monitoring your time spent on projects makes it easier to pinpoint and then correct inefficiencies. To track time spent, you can use a daily organizer, a plain notepad, or even one of the many time management software programs available.

• Plan a homework and study schedule that maximizes good results and minimizes anxiety.

• Set high but realistic academic standards. Consider all of your obligations when setting goals for the amount of time you think you'll be able to spend completing an assignment. Overestimating or underestimating time spent leads quickly to inefficiencies in time management.

• Study every day. You might study a lot on some days and less on others. No matter how much you study, make sure to study *something* every day. That way, you'll always be moving toward your goals.

- Use a calendar to record significant dates, such as tests and deadlines for term papers. The calendar will help you make sure you leave enough time to prepare for the test or complete the assignment.
- Plan for studying and completing assignments as far ahead of the deadline as possible. Making the most efficient use of your time involves allowing sufficient time for those unexpected events that can occur. Include deadlines for smaller tasks to help stay on track for finishing a big project.
- Plan to work on your assignments when activities that you'd like to participate in aren't also scheduled. That way, your mind will be free to concentrate more fully on your studies.
- Keep your study area organized and uncluttered.
- Complete each task at hand. Don't shuffle from one project to another without finishing the current task.
- Learn to say no to people when you don't have time to fulfill their requests.
- Use your precious leisure time as a reward for getting course work done on time and meeting your study goals.

> This is a bigger assignment than I thought. I'm glad I didn't put it off.

I always seem to be studying at the last minute. How can I avoid cramming?

The trouble with cramming, as you probably already know, is that it doesn't work. When you cram for a test, you don't really learn. Most of the information crammed into your brain in that short time disappears within hours. By the time of the test, your brain can be so tired that it can't retrieve the information you've only recently crammed into it. As a result, you "blank out" and are unable to answer questions you might be able to answer easily under other circumstances.

When faced with an examination for which you're unprepared, your best course of action is to stay calm and focused. Double-check with a classmate about the format of the test and where and when it will be given. Use your textbook to create a master study outline. Focus on chapter headings, summaries, highlighted words, formulas, definitions, and the first and last sentences of every para-

> When you aren't prepared for a test, staying calm is your most important asset.

graph. Write key points and an outline of each chapter on some notebook paper.

When you finish outlining, review your class notes and handouts. Then make some "must-know" flash cards outlining what you believe to be the most important information. Flip through these flash cards and review your outline repeatedly until you're too tired to continue. Then sleep a minimum of 4 hours. Make sure to awaken at least 1 hour before the test and review your outline and flip through your flash cards again. Be sure to wear a watch to manage your time efficiently during the test.

I can't find a place to study that I like. How do I choose the best study area for me?

You can study anywhere you choose but you should make sure that the study area affords comfort and an opportunity to accomplish a significant amount of work. Although many students say they study best when they're surrounded by distractions, they probably study least efficiently in those situations. Keep these points in mind when selecting an area to study:

• Select a place where you can concentrate deeply for an extended period.

• Remove distractions or at least reduce their effect as much as possible. For instance, if you must study in a room with a television, at least keep the sound turned down.

• Review the concepts you've studied, even during such everyday activities as getting dressed, eating meals, and driving home.

• Stimulate your thinking by studying in groups, talking with friends about the topic under study, or joining an interdisciplinary study group.

You can concentrate more efficiently when you aren't distracted by TV or your friends at the next table.

I have trouble concentrating. How can I concentrate better?

When you have several subjects to study in a day with more than one deadline looming, it's easy to become distracted and lose your concentration. When you lose concentration, you make less effective use of valuable study time. To help stay focused, keep these tips in mind:

• Alternate the order of the subjects you study during the day to add variety to your study. Try alternating your studies between the courses you find most interesting and those you find least interesting.

• Approach your studies with enthusiasm, sincerity, and determination.

• As soon as you've decided to study, begin immediately. Don't let anything interfere with your thought processes after you've begun.

• Concentrate on accomplishing one thing at a time, to the exclusion of everything else.

• Don't try to do two things at once, such as studying and watching television or conversing with friends.

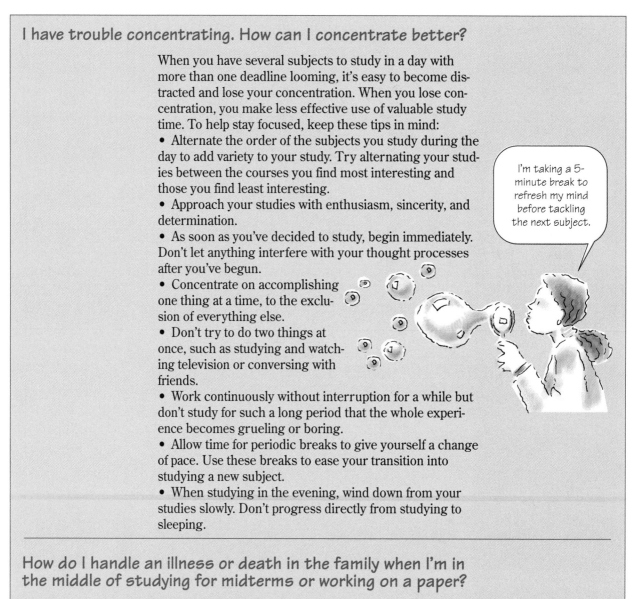

I'm taking a 5-minute break to refresh my mind before tackling the next subject.

• Work continuously without interruption for a while but don't study for such a long period that the whole experience becomes grueling or boring.

• Allow time for periodic breaks to give yourself a change of pace. Use these breaks to ease your transition into studying a new subject.

• When studying in the evening, wind down from your studies slowly. Don't progress directly from studying to sleeping.

How do I handle an illness or death in the family when I'm in the middle of studying for midterms or working on a paper?

Your own illness, an illness or death in your family, or other stressful events may cause you to fall behind in your studies. To clear the way for your return to classes following such an event, follow these tips for getting back on track quickly:

• Notify your instructors as soon as you know that you'll be missing class. Ask for upcoming assignments so you can continue with at least minimal studying for topics being covered in your absence.

- Make arrangements to study at home, if possible. Using the Internet for research and communications can be invaluable for completing assignments and discussing issues with instructors and classmates over e-mail. A growing number of educational institutions are using streaming video and other advanced technologies to make it easier for students to "attend" classes from home.
- Lighten your load at home and, to the extent possible, at school as well. Cut out all nonessential duties so you don't overwhelm yourself during times of physical or emotional stress.

> In case of a personal problem, find out if your institution offers take-at-home classes using the Internet.

I'm returning to school after raising a family. Help!!!

Adults returning to a school environment after a prolonged absence typically find that they need to be more attentive about their study habits than do their younger classmates. An adult student might have forgotten much of the material learned years ago and the material itself might have changed. The typical adult student may also have a number of other responsibilities, including children, a spouse, a home, and a career.

When you return to school, it's important to communicate to everyone in your family and at work how your life is changing and how those changes might affect them. For example, if you normally fix dinner every Thursday night, you might let your partner know that the family should count on having pizza because anatomy lab is on Thursday night. Likewise, if you usually stay late at work,

> Balancing work, school, and family may be difficult but it's worth the effort.

you'll need to tell your supervisors that you need to leave on time on Thursdays.

As a returning student, it's doubly important for you to surround yourself with people who will support you and pull some extra weight around the house and at work when a big assignment looms. Remind them that the situation is temporary and that you'll celebrate with them each time a semester ends and you get a bit of a break.

I'm overloaded with writing assignments. How do I handle a writing assignment quickly and easily?

Writing research papers and nursing care plans are common assignments for nursing students. The prospect of having to write an in-depth research paper or extensive plan of care can seem daunting at the least or, at worst, overwhelming to even the most competent student. To improve your efficiency at completing a writing assignment, follow these tips:

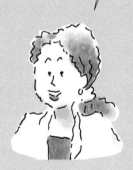

Take each writing assignment one step at a time to ensure success.

• When given a choice, select a topic or patient care condition you're familiar with and then adapt the topic or condition to your strengths.
• Write an outline about the topic or condition, and assess what information you'll need and the feasibility of gathering that information within the time frame of the project.
• Using a library and other resources, prepare a list of books and articles you need to complete the assignment. Then gather those materials.
• Refine your topic and refocus your thesis as indicated.
• Rewrite your outline, leaving room in the margins and between the lines to make notes.
• Maintain a list of the sources you use. Write down the source, author's name, and page number on which the information appears.
• Write your first draft and compile a bibliography.
• Create your final draft. Make sure that you've satisfied the teacher's specific requirements for the paper. Finally, proofread your paper for spelling and grammatical errors.

I never know what my instructor's tests will cover. It seems there's always stuff on the tests that wasn't covered in the textbook. What do I do?

Some instructors give their lecture material more weight than textbook material when composing a test. If you assume that a test will cover mostly information in the textbook, you could be shocked when test time rolls around and the test covers more of the lecture material than textbook material. To get the most from your lecture notes, you need to keep up with the teacher and maintain as active a role as possible. Here's how:

• Listen carefully to the instructor and take frequent notes.

• Try to identify what the instructor thinks is important. When an instructor repeats information or seems more enthusiastic about certain material, take it as a cue that the information is important.

• Understand that a lecture attempts to provide information for you to learn and apply to real-life situations. You need to dig into each lecture and take knowledge from it, as opposed to letting the lecture passively give you knowl-

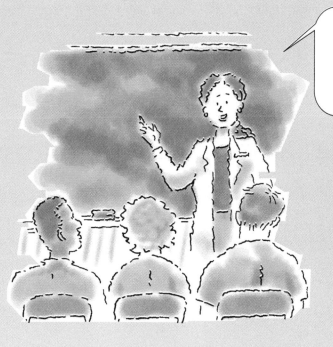

edge. The more active a role you play, the greater the learning that results.

• Attend as many lectures as possible. Never skip a lecture unless doing so is unavoidable. Even then, ask a classmate for a copy of her notes for that particular lecture. Most students don't mind giving copies of their notes for isolated lectures. After all, they may need to use your notes for a lecture they might miss someday.

• Sit in the front two or three rows of the class so you can see and hear the instructor well. This position also reduces the number of distractions between you and the instructor and allows you to concentrate more efficiently.

My notes are a mess. I never know what to take notes on and when I should or shouldn't take notes verbatim. How can I improve my note taking?

When taking notes in class, keep in mind that your objective should be to use the notes as a way of learning, understanding, and preparing material for later study. The system you use for taking notes should vary according to the lecturer's style and the information being covered. Follow these tips to get the most out of your classroom notes:

• Avoid taking notes verbatim. Record only essential ideas and summaries of important concepts.

• Record important ideas using short key terms. Organize these ideas logically, according to how your brain most efficiently processes information. For instance, if you're primarily a visual learner, you might organize your notes in a flowchart. If you tend to learn best in sequences, you might number your notes in an outline form.

• Write notes in your own words — not the instructor's. That way, you'll be more likely to remember the material later.

• Be sure to copy all charts, diagrams, and graphs that the instructor draws on the chalkboard during class. You'll use these graphic elements later to reinforce and clarify your notes.

• Write legibly. The best notes in the world won't help you study later if you can't read your own handwriting. Take notes with the understanding that you'll need to read or rewrite them later. You don't have to use perfect grammar, and routine spelling errors are perfectly acceptable. Even

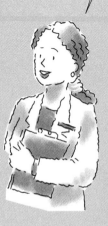

When taking class notes, leave plenty of space on the paper to fill in gaps and clarify points later.

so, do whatever you can to keep your notes neat and legible.

• Leave blank spaces throughout your notes to make comments in later. You can then return to your notes and add clarifying statements based on readings in the textbook or fill in information you might have missed in the lecture.

• Organize your notes by putting the date and name of the class at the top of the page.

• Be flexible and creative when taking notes. If drawing an arrow from notes on one page to notes on the previous page seems to make sense and will help you learn the material, then by all means, draw the arrow. Let your notes work for you; avoid being rigid with note-taking techniques. Fit the way you take notes to the content — not the other way around.

I find that when I get to class, I'm not really prepared for what we're covering. How can I prepare better for class?

If you don't read an assigned chapter, you might have a difficult time following a lecture based on that chapter. To make sure you're properly prepared when you attend class, follow these guidelines:

• Complete assignments from the previous class, especially textbook readings.

• Keep one step ahead. Don't wait to hear the lecture before you read the chapter on the topic.

• Before class, review notes from the previous lecture as well as the assigned reading for that class. Then you can connect what you learn in this lecture to what you already know.

• Bring your textbook to class. Your teacher may refer to it. Use sticky notes to mark specific pages referred to by the instructor.

• Bring your notes from your textbook assignment. You may decide to add lecture notes directly to the notes you took for your textbook assignment.

• Arrive on time. Teachers commonly make important announcements during the first few minutes of class. Missing those first few minutes could put you at a distinct disadvantage for upcoming tests and assignments.

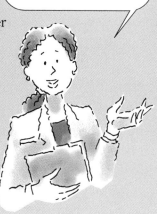

Forget audiotaping lectures. Listening well and taking good notes are more efficient.

- Choose a location that allows you to concentrate more easily.
- Wait before asking a question. The instructor may answer the question in the course of the lecture. Write your questions down so you don't forget them during the lecture.
- When in doubt, ask for an example. Examples are usually easier to understand than abstract explanations of important concepts.
- Listen to the questions your classmates ask and the insights they give into the topic being discussed.
- Don't use a tape recorder unless you must. Tape recorders double the amount of time you spend listening to your instructor.
- Quiz yourself immediately after the lecture. Take a minute or two to summarize what was just covered in class to identify weaknesses in your memory of the material. Then review your notes and the textbook to fill in gaps in your memory or to answer questions that arise out of your self-quiz immediately after class.

Tests scare me to death. I get so anxious before a test that I can't study right. How can I avoid becoming so anxious before a test?

A little worrying can be a good thing. Research indicates that mild anxiety sharpens a person's level of alertness and enhances problem-solving abilities. Being more than a little anxious, though, can reduce your ability to recall information, a critical task for taking a test. To reduce your level of anxiety before a test:

- Prepare well in advance. Avoid last minute cramming. Don't go without sleep the night before the test. Stop studying an hour or so before the test to relax and compose yourself.
- Worry only about what is real. You have cause to worry only if you didn't study for the test. If you studied and you're prepared, worrying about what could be on the test or how well you'll do will only make you more anxious and decrease the likelihood of success.

> If I get a little anxious before a big test, I try to stay focused and relaxed with slow, deep breaths.

SNAP

- Know the time and place of the test and what articles or implements you need to bring.
- Arrive a little early to organize yourself before class.
- Don't talk about the test with classmates immediately before the test if you know that doing so will make you worry more. Feeding into group paranoia about a test won't help anyone, including you.
- Read over the test and plan your approach. For example, determine early which questions are worth the most points and how long you plan to spend on each question.
- If a question is unclear, don't hesitate to ask for clarification.
- Try to relax yourself during the test. Take several slow, deep breaths. Concentrate on your breathing.
- Pay attention to the test, not to other people in the room. Try not to wonder about how the student next to you is doing or whether you'll score as well as you hope. Instead, focus on taking the test and answering all questions as well as you can.

I'm taking a course I hate with an instructor I don't understand. It's really frustrating. Any tips?

Anger, anxiety, and a lack of confidence in your skills and knowledge can impair recall and ultimately lead to lower test scores. So it's as important to prepare your emotions for a test as it is to prepare your mind with all the information you need to remember. Here's how:

- Study the course work so you're sure that you know it well. There is nothing like properly preparing for a test to bolster your self-confidence. If you feel confident about passing, you'll lose some of your anxiety about the test. However, don't become so overconfident that you become careless.
- Minimize anxiety by studying in the same room where the test will be administered, if possible. Sit in a favorite seat. Do some homework there. Get familiar with the surroundings. The more familiar your surroundings during the test, the more relaxed you'll feel.
- Before entering the testing room, make a concerted effort to rid yourself of the anger you might be feeling. Identify the angry feelings, recognize that the feelings will interfere with your more immediate goal of obtaining a good

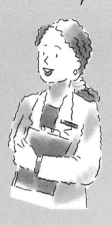

Give yourself a pat on the back when you've prepared properly for a test.

test score, and then tell yourself that it's okay to leave the anger behind you.

• Know that sometimes it's a good idea to postpone a test. For example, if you're ill or in pain from an injury, postponing the test might make good sense. Always check with the instructor to determine whether you'll lose points for delaying the test. Never postpone a test because of fear or anxiety about the test. Doing so only delays the inevitable.

• Alleviate test-taking anxiety through positive reinforcement. A little positive reinforcement can serve as a reminder that you're prepared for the test and an incentive for feeling confident in your knowledge.

I keep making silly mistakes on tests. I know the material but I get the questions wrong. How can I avoid making silly mistakes?

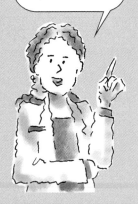

To avoid making mistakes, always read the question twice.

Whether you're taking an essay, multiple-choice, or short-answer test, be sure to read all instructions and all questions carefully. If you make a mistake in reading the instructions, you could jeopardize your grade for the entire examination. Likewise, be sure to read each test question carefully. Misreading a test question can cause you to:

• incorrectly analyze what the question is asking

• overlook important cue words, such as *early, late, unsafe,* or *inappropriate*

• read information into a question that isn't part of the question.

To avoid misreading a question or reading into it, restate the question in your own words.

I just hate multiple-choice questions. I have a hard time figuring out the "best" option. What strategies can I use to take multiple-choice tests more effectively?

For a multiple-choice test, try first to answer the question without looking at the options. Then eliminate each option that includes new information not stated in the question. Determine what the question is asking and which of the options are possible answers. When you find it hard to choose between options in a multiple-choice test, try these tips:

- Eliminate all options you *know* are incorrect. Focus on the options you're unsure about.
- Identify the global response. A global response is a more general statement that may also include correct ideas from other options. Depending on the question, the most comprehensive or generalized option is probably a better answer than an option that may be correct but is more specific or limited.
- Eliminate similar options. Because there can be only one best option in most multiple-choice tests, eliminate both options if they say essentially the same thing or include the same idea. In those cases, neither could be the correct answer.
- Look for similar words used in the question and in the options. If you find a word, feeling, or behavior in the question *and* in one of the options, the option containing the same word, feeling, or behavior as the question is probably the correct option.

> Take a step-by-step approach to multiple-choice questions.

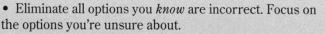

It's the essay test I hate. I hate writing and always come off looking like an idiot. How can I take an essay test better?

To take an essay test, first read through the entire test. Select the questions you feel most capable of answering, and figure out about how much time you can spend on each one. Next to each question, note the number of minutes you plan to spend on it.

On a separate sheet, write down the facts you're most unsure about and that you think you'll be most likely to forget. For example, you might write down key dates, definitions, or conditions.

For each essay question, create a brief, logical outline of everything you can remember about the topic. If you haven't kept up with class, you probably won't be able to offer an interpretation of the topic but you can at least organize your thoughts and try to provide a rational framework for all the facts you can remember. Be sure to write neatly and spell terms correctly. When you finish, read your answer from beginning to end and correct all glaring spelling, grammatical, and punctuation errors.

> To recall key facts, write them down as soon as you can. Then use the fact sheet to answer the questions.

I tend to spend too much time on questions I can't answer, and then don't have enough time left to answer the ones I know. How can I plan my test-taking time better?

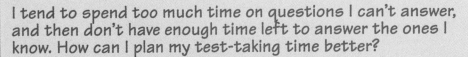

When in doubt, follow your instincts. They're usually correct.

When faced with a multiple-choice or short-answer test for which you're unprepared, "triage" the questions first. "Triaging" allows you to distinguish between questions you can answer quickly and those that will take a while.

To "triage" a multiple-choice or short-answer test, go through the entire test and immediately answer every question to which you know the answer. Place a question mark next to questions whose answer you think you might be able to figure out, and place an X by questions that completely stump you.

After answering all the easy-to-answer questions, return to the questions you identified with a question mark. Give yourself a minute or two to arrive at an answer but avoid spending too much time on a single question. If you can't arrive at an acceptable answer within a couple of minutes, skip the question and move on.

After answering all of the more difficult questions, you can try to answer all questions marked with an X. If you have even a hint about a question, think about it for a minute and give it the best answer you can. Remember that your first instinct for an answer is probably the correct one. Pay attention to that instinct and follow it as much as possible. Then, during whatever time remains in the examination period, guess at the other answers. Try never to leave answers blank.

Some tests call for you to write definitions of terms. I generally know the meaning of a term but I usually can't put it on paper clearly enough. Any tips?

Knowing in your mind what a term means and being able to write it clearly on paper are two different things, as you well know. Most instructors don't want you to spit back a textbook definition of a key term; they want to see whether you understand the term and can apply it to a clinical situation. Here are some tips to use to show the instructor you can do just that:

• Before writing the definition, jot down a few key words that relate to the term you're trying to define. For instance, if you're defining *mitochondria,* you might jot down *energy, intracellular, organelle,* and *ATP synthesis.* After this mini-brainstorming session, use the terms to form a definition in your own words.

- Keep your definition brief. Remember that your instructor isn't looking for a 3-page essay, just a sense that you're familiar with the term and have a clear understanding of its meaning.
- For each term, consider writing an example of how the term might be applied to the clinical area. For instance, you might provide this example for *pronation:* "For instance, when taking a radial pulse, you should have the patient pronate his hand." (By the way, "for instance" and "for example" are great ways to start the sentence.)

> Keep your definitions brief and offer an example of using the term in the clinical area.

Sometimes I just get stumped on a question. What can I do when that happens?

You'll no doubt have times when you can't answer a question because you don't have enough time or information. When that happens, any of these strategies will get you back on track and "unstump" you:

- Ask the teacher to clarify or rephrase a question, or try rephrasing the question yourself.
- Come back to the question later.
- Visualize where in the textbook or your notes the information was located. Try to recall the time and place you last reviewed the fact. Try to reconstruct the information using what you know.
- Start writing. When you start writing, other ideas will most likely come to mind.
- If you can't answer a question as asked, try to think of a related question or a more general question about the topic, either of which might provide enough of a clue about the actual question that you'll be able to answer the question correctly.
- If you're short of time on an essay question, write "Short of time" and finish your answer in outline form.
- When you're stumped on an essay question, try answering it using plain common sense and not specific classroom material. Imagine you've never taken the course

> Can't answer an essay question? Replace it with one you *can* answer.

at all. How would you respond? Putting yourself into another frame of mind might be enough to spark a recollection about the information being tested and give you something with which to answer the question.

- If you're taking an essay test, you might replace a question you can't answer at all with a related one that you *can* answer. Your answer must let the teacher know that you know you aren't answering the question asked; otherwise, it might seem as if you didn't understand the question or weren't willing to answer it. Replacing one question with another shows that you've gained relevant and valuable knowledge in the course even if that knowledge isn't being tested on this particular examination.

Yes, obstacles can crop up. But believe in your ability to handle them. You can do it, I know you can!

Part 3 Special skills

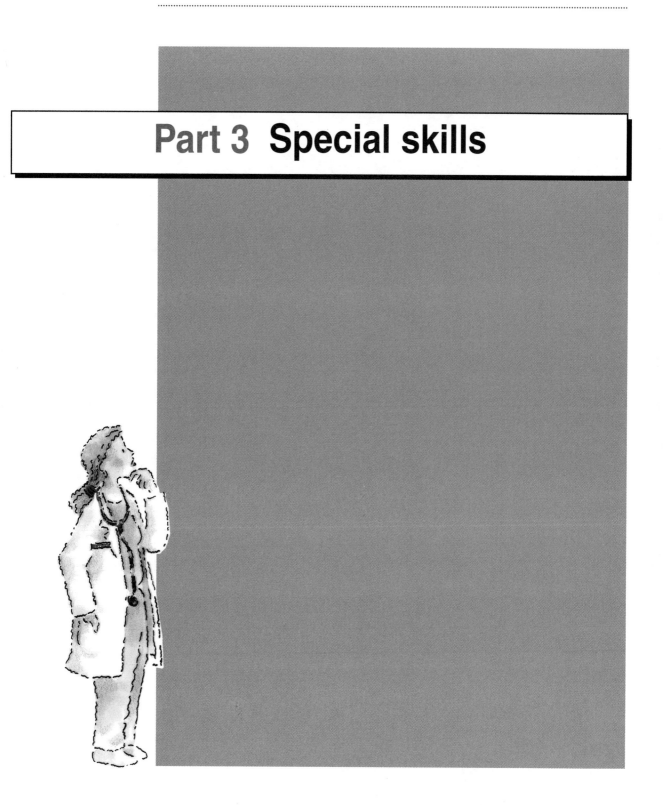

9

Writing a paper

Just the facts

In this chapter, you'll learn:

♦ what resources are available for researching a paper and how to use them effectively

♦ how to structure a paper, including creating an introduction, a body, and a conclusion

♦ why the first draft of a paper is only one step on the way to a finished paper

♦ why editing and polishing the paper involves not just spellchecking, but proofreading thoroughly.

Elements of a paper

An assignment to "write a paper" for a class may mean writing an essay, in which the writer attempts to make a persuasive point; a report that explains the main facts of a particular book, article, or other text; or a research paper, in which the writer brings many different sources together to discuss a particular topic.

In all these cases, however, the paper contains three main elements: an introduction, body, and conclusion. Although certain assignments — such as writing a memoir, short story, or other narrative — can call for a more fluid structure, the introduction, body, and conclusion form the basis for most written assignments. Depending on the length and complexity of your assignment, the paper may also include, in the order in which it appears:

• title page
• table of contents
• bibliography and other appendices.

Introductory material

Introductory material for a paper can include a title page, table of contents, and introductory text. The title page usually contains your name, the paper's title, the name of the course and instructor, and the date. The instructor may request information to be formatted in a particular way, so be sure your title page conforms to those specifications.

Which chapter first?

The table of contents, which follows the title page in long assignments, gives page numbers for all the elements included in the paper. This element provides an easy reference point if the paper contains several chapters.

Allow me to introduce myself

The introduction of the paper contains a brief explanation of where the text is headed. It should get your reader's attention and explain the point of the discussion. It should also contain the paper's thesis, a statement that encapsulates what you're writing about. If you're trying to persuade the reader, the thesis outlines the main point you intend to make.

Not always written first

Although the introduction appears at the beginning of the paper, it isn't necessarily the first part of the paper to be written. The introduction may consist of only 5% to 10% of the total amount of words in your final paper, but it takes thought and time. Sometimes, if you're stuck on the introduction, skip it and work on it again after you've written some of the rest of the paper.

Your introduction may begin with your thesis statement, an unusual fact, or even a story.

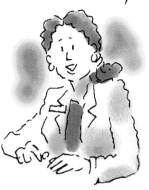

It was a dark and stormy night...

Although your introduction can begin with a thesis statement, many other, more intriguing ways to start your paper are possible, including:
• posing a question or problem
• describing a dramatic incident
• citing unusual facts or figures
• setting a scene
• telling a brief story.

Advice from the experts

Weighting the parts of a paper

Before writing a paper, you may want to gauge roughly how many pages should be devoted to the introduction, body of the paper, and conclusion. Unless your instructor provides other directions, use these guidelines for weighting the various parts of a typical paper:

Element	Percentage
Introduction	5% to 15%
Body	70% to 90%
Conclusion	5% to 15%

Body

The body of the paper, which supports the thesis, makes up the bulk of the paper's length. (See *Weighting the parts of a paper.*) The body of the paper makes your point, gives facts, and cites supporting research. In the body, you may want to start by writing background and historical information on the topic. Explain special terms or phrases used in the text. The body is also where you present arguments against your thesis and then defend your statement.

Closing material

Your paper should close as dramatically and effectively as it opens. After a strong conclusion, your paper may make use of a bibliography or appendixes to support the material contained in the body.

Conclusion

The key element of the closing material — the conclusion — should convey a fitting sense of ending your discussion. A simple summary of main points is rarely enough for a conclusion; instead, a conclusion should leave the reader with something for further thought or consideration. Effective strategies to employ in a conclusion include:
- citing a relevant quotation
- asking a pertinent question
- calling for action to support your point

• including a final example or story that illustrates your point.

Bibliography

The bibliography explains where you obtained your information and gives credit to the people whose research or quotes are cited in your paper. In general, each entry in a bibliography lists — alphabetically by the author's last name — the author's name; name of the article, journal, or book where you found the information; date of publication; city of publication; and publisher's name.

When writing a conclusion, try to leave the reader with food for thought.

Appendices

An appendix contains information that supports your paper but is too lengthy to include or condense within the body of the paper. An appendix might consist of terms, photos, tables, charts, figures, or other supportive material pertinent to your thesis.

Approach to writing

After you've established the type of paper you're going to write and the elements it will contain, plan how to approach the task of writing. Here are the basic steps for producing a polished paper:
• Set a schedule.
• Choose a topic.
• Gather information.
• Evaluate the information.
• Organize the information.
• Write an outline.
• Write a first draft.
• Revise the initial draft.
• Edit and polish the paper.

Setting a schedule

Setting up a schedule for working on your paper will help you stay focused on your target and maintain a steady, effective writing and researching pace. To set up a schedule, use your school calendar and work backward from the due date. Mark the:

- date you need to begin research
- date you need to complete research
- time you need for writing the rough draft
- time you need for revising the paper
- due date for the entire paper.

Scope it out

Don't set out to write a 20-page paper when the instructor wants a 10-page paper, and don't write a 10-page paper when the instructor wants one twice as long. You can gauge the amount of work you'll need to write the paper in part by figuring out:

- how many pages the paper should be
- how much time you have to work on it
- how much research the instructor expects you to do
- how many references the instructor expects you to cite.

> Use the assigned page length to gauge how much work you'll need to do to complete the assignment.

Keep it manageable

Start early. Schedule your work in manageable pieces. Schedule time to do research and to gather the materials you need. Build delays into your schedule. A book you need may already be checked out of the library when you try to find it, or someone you want to interview may cancel the interview or be away on sabbatical at that time. In addition, schedule time to peruse the materials you gather. After compiling the material, evaluate it for usefulness.

Choosing a topic

How you choose a topic depends on your assignment: Your instructor may assign a topic or give you a list of topics from which to choose. Always choose a topic that stimulates your interest. If the assignment demands research, consider the availability of resources.

Ideas are everywhere

Keep in mind that the more narrow the topic, the more focused your writing process and your finished paper. It's easier to stay focused, for example, when writing about how to use a screwdriver than it is when describing how to use tools in general. Ideas for topics can come from a number of places, including:

- table of contents in a textbook
- class notes
- conversation or brainstorming with classmates
- other media, such as newspapers, television, or magazines.

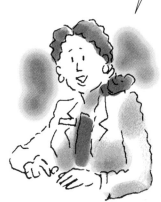

Thinking about your paper's title helps narrow your focus.

What's in a name?

When choosing your topic, think about what your thesis statement and title are going to be. You may want to leave the piece untitled until you finish the paper, but it helps to be thinking about a title even if it isn't used for the finished paper. A good title should be clear and catchy and not so obscure that the reader needs to make a mental jump or know an inside joke to understand what the paper is about.

Gathering information

Various sources and methods for gathering information are available, depending on the scope of the project and your access to those sources. Sources of information can include:

- library resources
- experts in the field
- surveys
- online resources
- objective observations
- personal experiences.

Gotta luuuuuuv the library

Your first stop in your quest for information should be the library. Look up your topic in the card catalog or computer system. (See *Understanding call numbers,* page 190.) Look through the specialized indexes available in the library's reference section, including *Reader's Guide to Periodical Literature*, which lists titles and subjects of articles published in magazines and journals. Other reference books include encyclopedias and specialized dictionaries. Libraries also keep maps and pamphlets that may be useful.

The reference librarian is an excellent source of information, not only for guidance during the course of your research but also for guidance about how to use the library.

Dr. Iman Expert, PhD

Depending on the nature of your topic, you may want to speak to professors elsewhere in the school, experts in the field, or anyone else with relevant knowledge on the subject. Discussions with experts in the field, though commonly difficult to schedule, can prove helpful in narrowing your search for information and for clarifying your topic. If you need to interview an expert in the field or another individual during your research, be prepared before conducting the interview. Write out all the questions you want to ask, ranking each on its importance and relevance to your research topic. Ask the most relevant questions first.

Keep in mind that in an interview — whether it's a telephone interview or face to face — you're in charge of the interview and are responsible for steering the conversation to meet your needs. If the interviewee agreed to spend 30 minutes with you, discuss the important topics on your list first. Avoid chatting about unrelated topics, such as the weather or favorite vacation spots. Doing so could cause you to lose the opportunity to ask key questions.

Whenever possible, audiotape the interview for later reference. Be sure to ask the interviewee's permission to let you tape the interview. You may want to do this when

Do you mind if I tape this interview? I want to make sure everything I write is accurate.

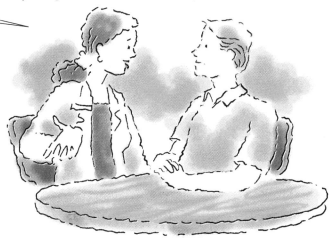

Advice from the experts

Understanding call numbers

Most libraries follow one or more systems of call numbers for classifying and storing resources. This table outlines the Dewey Decimal System and the Library of Congress system for call numbers.

Subject	Dewey Decimal	Library of Congress
General works	000	A
Philosophy and psychology	100, 150	B to BF
Religion	200	BL to BX
History	900	C to F
Geography	910	G
Social science	300	H
Political science	320	J
Law	340	K
Education	370	L
Music	780	M
Fine arts	700	N
Language	400	P
Literature	800	P
Natural science and mathematics	500, 510	Q
Medicine	610	R
Agriculture	630	S
Applied science and technology	600	T
Military and naval science	350	U to V
Bibliography	010	Z

setting up the meeting to avoid awkward moments at the time of the interview.

Using an audiotape to record the interview doesn't mean you don't need to take notes. A battery failure, failure to press the record button, or use of a damaged tape can result in partial or total loss of the interview. In those cases, your notes will be your only backup. When the audiotape functions properly, of course, you can use it to enhance your notes with exact quotes and to fill in gaps of information.

Surveying the landscape

In the survey, you'll ask the same questions of a number of subjects. You'll later compile the answers and perform calculations on the totals. For instance, you might calculate the percentage of all subjects who answered *Yes* to a particular question versus the percentage of subjects over age 25 who answered *Yes* to the question. The results of your survey can play a large role in your paper, depending on the relevance, reliability, and comprehensiveness of the data.

It's a mad, mad, mad, mad World Wide Web

Using a computer with access to the Internet, you can find a wealth of background material and reference works. Some libraries have facilities available for students to go online and search the World Wide Web section of the Internet for information. When using the Web to research a topic, carefully evaluate each piece of information for reliability. Just because something is on the Internet doesn't mean it's accurate. Use Internet information from reputable sources only. Then make sure you cite the information properly, including the address, site owner, and other available information according to the format required by your instructor.

I observe

Relying on your own observation is a highly subjective research tool. You may interpret an event in a different way than another person who experiences the same event. You can overcome your own subjectivity by taking notes and keeping a checklist when you begin making your observations. If you plan to observe a situation and write about it, such as analyzing behavior on the playground, keep a checklist of what you intend to observe for and take copious notes. Your notes and checklist will provide consistency and reliability to your findings.

I experience

Personal experiences may be useful in completing your assignment, but they often work best in conjunction with

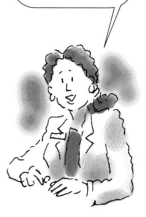

Keep copious notes when making observations you plan to cite in your paper.

more objective sources. Be sure to include personal experiences relevant to the assignment only, and make sure that the instructor considers personal experiences appropriate source material.

Organizing the information

Small index cards can be indispensable as you organize your information. Using one index card for each source, write key ideas from the source and the page numbers on which you found them. You'll use this information later to build your bibliography. Armed with a generous supply of index cards, you can begin sorting through the information you've obtained and judging sources on their reliability and relevance.

Basics

Start with the most general sources first, and then work your way to the more specific sources. Look for basic information about your topic so you can become familiar with the topic and build your knowledge from there. Take copious notes on the material. Transcribe quotes accurately, making sure you can attribute the quote to a source and enclose the quote in quotation marks. As an added measure, you might mark pertinent areas of information in the source material with colorful, removable paper notes.

Sorting through the chaos

As you begin to see repetition in the material, start sorting the index cards by topic or according to the part of the paper in which you think the information will appear — early, toward the middle, at the end. You can weed out redundant information and select the most helpful sources at this point.

Coding the cards by symbol or color is a useful method of staying organized. You can use colored dot stickers to color-code the cards or mark them with colored pens or symbols. Use an asterisk to indicate background information and an X to indicate counterpoint information.

Judging relevance

After gathering your materials, you may find that some of the resources are irrelevant to your paper. Perhaps the information is old or outdated. As a rule of thumb, avoid using sources older than 5 years. Always evaluate the information you've obtained for relevance and reliability.

For example, you may find that a source argues against your thesis but has no supporting information. Such information, even though you found it in a published source, may not be worth including in your paper.

On the other hand, you may find counterpoint information supported by documented facts. In such a case, you should include that argument in your paper. If the argument is so compelling as to weaken your thesis, you might want to reconsider the focus of your paper. It's better to examine arguments at an early, information-gathering stage than to struggle later to write a paper supported by a weak foundation.

> This information is irrelevant! Strike it from the paper!

About the author

The bias of an author can influence your writing, so try to distinguish unsupported personal opinion from thoughtful commentary. If the author criticizes or condemns without providing solid examples of what is meant, the information may not be useful to your paper. Remember as well that statistics cited in a source don't immediately make that source reliable; statistics can be manipulated as easily as words.

Primary colors

> Treat all statistics with that proverbial grain of salt. Just because someone says it's a "fact" doesn't make it factual.

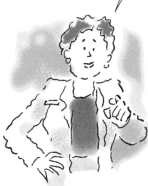

Determine whether your sources are primary or secondary. A primary source is the original document or first-hand account of an event. A secondary source is a restatement of what was said in a primary source. Bear in mind that a statement from a primary source may be taken out of context and published in a secondary source, where its meaning becomes obscured. If possible, work from primary sources rather than relying on secondary sources.

Writing an outline

After assembling your information, begin outlining your paper. As you develop your topic, use outlining and charting methods to consolidate the notes you made on index cards. In the outline, state the theme or thesis of the paper as your introduction, and then write a brief conclusion. This draft of a conclusion will help you stay focused on your theme.

Then, even if you won't use a title page, table of contents, or bibliography in your first draft, incorporate these elements into your outline as one-line entries.

Order! Order!

How you arrange your outline headings depends on how you intend to organize the paper. Keep in mind that the outline can be adjusted as necessary as you write the paper. The outline serves as an organizational guide, not a set of commands.

Writing the first draft

The first draft of your paper is where you sketch out your introduction, the text of the paper, and the conclusion. As you write, keep your audience in mind. Knowing for whom you're writing helps you maintain a consistent tone and voice. If you're writing strictly for your instructor, keep a mental image of the instructor in your mind as you write.

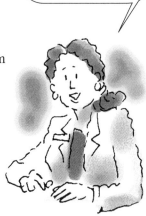

The first draft sets the stage for the final paper.

If you have access to a computer, you may want to write directly on the computer, remembering to save a copy of the information on a floppy diskette or other backup format. Using a computer allows you to easily rearrange or reword material without having to retype the paper. Some people, however, prefer to write the first draft using longhand.

Just put it down

Once you begin writing the first draft, don't slow yourself down by trying to polish your writing. Just get the ideas down on paper. For instance, don't waste time in the first draft trying to write a perfect introduction — just put some kind of introduction on paper. You can revise later. Do the same with the body of the paper and the conclusion.

Let the outline be your guide

Use your outline as a guide. If you wanted to organize the paper in a certain way — for instance, a chronological sequence — stick with that format unless you determine as you write that the format isn't working. As you write, keep track of footnotes and bibliographic references.

Your mind continues to work on your paper even when you're not. Rest and let your mind work its magic.

Now, put it away

After writing the first draft, put the paper away for a little while. Even when you're not working on your paper, your brain is working on it and may suddenly give you exactly the introduction you need or the closing argument you've been looking for at times when you least expect it. Write these thoughts on paper, and then refer to them later when revising the first draft.

Temporarily setting aside the paper also allows you to reread the paper with a more critical eye. When you return to the paper, typographic errors and organizational changes you need to make will almost jump off the page at you.

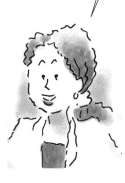

Revising the paper

After thinking about your paper for a little while, start writing the second draft. Allow yourself to make dramatic changes, moving chunks of text within the body of the paper as you shape the paper toward its final form.

Take precautions

Reorganizing your paper is less labor-intensive if it's done on computer. Just remember to save the revised file with a new filename so your original will remain intact. If later want to revert to the original organization, you can open the original file and copy-and-paste the appropriate sections. Keep revising your paper until all the pieces are in place in exactly the sequence you want them.

Let's see, that's 87 drafts of the same paper. Think that's enough? I certainly do!

How many drafts?

There's no fixed rule for how many times a paper should be revised. The idea is to revise your paper until you feel comfortable with the way it reads and what it says — while still handing it in on time. Remember, you're aiming to write the best paper possible. It may take several drafts to get there.

How does it flow?

At each new draft, reevaluate your work. Read the entire paper aloud. Hearing what you've written will help you quickly zero in on trouble spots. Pay particular attention to:
• organization. After moving text around, does it still make sense? Does the overall organization seem logical and clear?
• paragraph structure. Does each paragraph have a major idea and a topic sentence? Are the transitions from one paragraph to the next logical and coherent?
• sentence flow. Does each sentence within each paragraph lead logically and smoothly to the next?

> The paper looks good to me. Now's the time for someone else to read it with a critical eye.

The home stretch

After you've completed the body of the paper, create the missing pieces: title page, table of contents (leaving page numbers blank until the final edit), bibliography, and appendixes, if any. Then let someone else read the paper to find flaws in spelling, grammar, sentence construction, organization, logic, and other criteria the teacher may use to judge the paper. Don't automatically accept their comments and corrections as totally correct, however. You're the final judge.

Polishing the paper

After you're comfortable that the paper is close to its final form, it's time to polish. When polishing, ask yourself:
• Did I spellcheck the document?
• Did I verify words the spellchecker didn't understand?
• Do I always have a singular verb for a singular subject and a plural verb for a plural subject?
• Is there a period or other punctuation mark at the end of every sentence?
• Is there a single space only between sentences? Nearly all computer programs add a slight bit of space automatically after each period, making two spaces unnecessary and leaving too large a gap. Use two spaces between sentences only if the instructor requests it or if you're working on a typewriter rather than a computer.
• Is my use of terms consistent? Did I write *congestive heart failure* in one paragraph and *heart failure* in another?

Advice from the experts

Visual appeal

Some papers are easier to read than others because they have more white space around the text. White space gives the eye room to roam around without making the reader feel constrained.

To make a paper easier to review, use an unjustified, or ragged, right margin. Keep the left margin at least 1" (2.5 cm). Use 1½ or double spacing between the lines rather than single-spacing; double-spacing provides room in which the instructor can write comments.

• Does the tone of the paper remain consistent through-out?

• Is the type size large enough to be comfortable to read? (See *Visual appeal*.)

• Does the paper and the way it's presented look polished and professional?

Consult the experts

In formatting a research paper, you don't have to start from scratch. Your instructor may give you guidelines to follow, or you can consult style manuals available in the reference section of the library. These style manuals can help clarify questions about grammar, spelling, specialized terms and acronyms, and industry standards for style. Common editorial tools at your disposal include:

• general dictionaries

• specialized dictionaries — for example, medical or bio-logical dictionaries

• a thesaurus, which lists synonyms, antonyms, slang, and related words

• English grammar and usage guides

• editorial style guides such as the *Publication Manual of the American Psychological Association* or the *Chicago Manual of Style*.

Always proofread your work before handing it in.

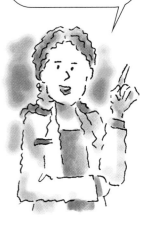

It pays to proofread

After you've edited your paper and made corrections, take another small break before proofreading. If you don't give yourself a break, you may not read as closely because you've seen the text many times before and you know what it's supposed to say. When proofreading:

• pay particular attention to weak areas, such as punctuation or capitalization
• read slowly and aloud, if possible, pronouncing each word and pausing for punctuation
• when you use a word that you don't generally use or are at all unsure about its meaning, look it up in the dictionary.

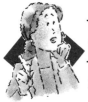

Quick quiz

1. In a bibliography, references are usually arranged:
   A. chronologically by the date of publication.
   B. alphabetically by the title of the book or article.
   C. alphabetically by the author's last name.
Answer: C. References in a bibliography are usually ordered alphabetically by the author's last name.

2. In a long paper, the table of contents should follow immediately after the:
   A. title page.
   B. introduction.
   C. first appendix.
Answer: A. The table of contents, which provides page numbers for all the elements included in the paper, follows the title page in long assignments.

3. A firsthand account of an event is considered a:
   A. primary source.
   B. secondary source.
   C. tertiary source.
Answer: A. A primary source is the original document or firsthand account of an event.

Scoring

☆☆☆   If you answered all three questions correctly, superb! Spectacular! Stupendous! You're our primary source for help in writing a paper!

☆☆   If you answered two questions correctly, congratulations! We'll call on you for help in finding Internet sources for a research paper!

☆   If you answered fewer than two questions correctly, don't fret. You're our favorite secondary source for editorial style questions.

Coping with math

Just the facts

In this chapter, you'll learn:

◆ how problem-solving skills can help a person succeed at math

◆ which health care skills involve math

◆ why increasing your math vocabulary can help make many math problems easier

◆ why cooperative learning makes math more enjoyable and easier to learn

◆ why estimating and guessing are valuable math skills.

Overcoming math anxiety

Few other subjects elicit as much fear, anxiety, and concern as math. Many people find the number-oriented language of math strange and foreign. Others had unpleasant experiences with math as young students. Overcoming math anxiety can be a tough job, but working through this chapter can give you an excellent start.

Why study math?

Math is hard to escape. Many people think that after high school, they wouldn't have to deal with math anymore, or at least only a little. The problem is, math keeps showing up. For example, health care professionals need to be competent in math to handle such situations as:
• measuring solutions for procedures
• figuring dosages
• converting pounds to kilograms for weights

No matter where you go in life, you'll meet up with math. Let's learn it *now!*

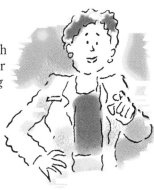

- determining I.V. drip rates
- developing department budgets
- scheduling staff assignments.

Dispelling math myths

Many people carry around a series of beliefs involving math that just aren't true. If you can shake off these myths, you'll probably have an easier time succeeding at math. Let's look at just a few of the many math myths you might encounter.

Math is based on problem solving.

Myth 1: I'm just no good at math

Do you consider yourself a problem-solver? Do you like to succeed? If so, you probably have a lot more potential for math than you thought. Many people consider math an area that they're just "no good at." In particular, many women have been trained to believe that math is a subject for men. They develop low expectations for themselves and write off math entirely.

However, math is based on solving problems. Few people would claim to be poor problem-solvers, so why claim to be poor at math? Start putting those problem-solving skills to work.

Myth 2: I have a calculator, so I don't need to know math

Like any other computer, a calculator is only as good as the person operating it. It's true that if you have a calculator, you don't need to multiply 41 times 23 in your head. But a calculator is only a tool. Saying you don't need to know math because you own a tool used in math is equivalent to saying, "Now that I have a hammer, I don't need to know anything about carpentry."

A calculator can help you navigate many math problems, but you're still in charge. Think of a calculator as a computer to help you with math, not prevent you from learning math.

Myth 3: I'll never use math anyway, so why learn it?

This myth evolved out of the fact that math is commonly learned in isolation and without concrete application to everyday life. Yet mathematical concepts are used throughout everyday life. You'll use the math you learn now at home and throughout your career in health care.

For instance, learning about ratios and proportions will allow you to ensure that your patient is receiving the correct I.V. drug infusion dosage. Learning other math concepts will allow you to formulate budgets (not just at work but at home, too), determine the extent of injury in a burned patient, and perform a host of other tasks.

Succeeding in math class

If thinking about math makes you groan, thinking about sitting in a math class probably doesn't seem like a lot of fun either. But once again, there's no good reason why you can't succeed. With a few helpful hints, you'll soon feel at home in any math class.

The instructor as resource

Many people are reluctant to ask an instructor— especially a math instructor— for help. They may worry about looking foolish or about asking "dumb" questions. Remember, though, there is no such thing as a dumb question. If you need some help, ask for it. (See *Calling in a coach,* page 202.)

The textbook as resource

Math textbooks can be intimidating. They're often filled with formulas and equations that can confuse the eye and boggle the brain. A textbook is a learning tool, though, and with some help you can learn to use a math textbook to your advantage.

Practice the problems

Most math textbooks supply plenty of practice problems. Use them to your advantage. Solve lots of problems, doing one type of problem at a time. Practicing this way helps you see some of the underlying patterns of a concept or technique and helps you develop a feel for solving each type of problem. In addition, by imitating the steps in the book, you can become familiar with the type of problem you're working on and build a solid foundation for applying that knowledge to other problems.

Remember, your teacher is there to help you understand math concepts. When you need help, ask for it.

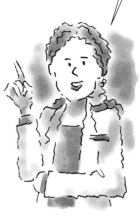

Advice from the experts

Calling in a coach

Your teacher isn't the only person you can turn to for help. Find a math mentor. Mentors can be almost anyone who understands math. You can also consider hiring a tutor, such as a teacher's aide or a math-proficient fellow student, or check the Internet for interactive practice problems, discussion boards, and online tutoring services. Remember, even professional athletes turn to special coaches for help when they need it. Don't tackle math alone; get help when you need it.

Put it in writing

Do each step on paper, not in your head. Even when you thoroughly understand a technique, force yourself to write down every step on paper. A concert pianist continues to practices the scales long after mastering far more difficult maneuvers. Writing out the steps helps you focus and gets your mind in the problem-solving groove.

Cut out carelessness

Get in the habit of reading *very* carefully; many errors are caused by misreading a problem rather than computing the math incorrectly. Even if you have to use your finger to follow each word, be sure to read the problem more carefully than you read anything else. It's *that* important.

Look for what's left out

If you don't understand the solution to a problem, the textbook author might have omitted some steps. Prepare a list of problems you can't work out, and discuss each with your teacher. Make certain you understand each type of problem you'll face on an examination.

Invest in your (math) future

Students sometimes think that the text assigned to a class is the only one they're allowed to use. However, supplementary sources can help clarify content in your main text and give you a greater variety of problems to solve. Find a resource with lots of examples and step-by-step solutions. See if the text includes proofs or derivations for the formulas it uses. Be aware that a different author may use a different notation system, so be sure to familiarize yourself with it.

Proper preparation for class

Math is a sequential subject. Nearly every concept is built on a previous one. Skipping assignments can quickly reduce your understanding of math in general. Set time aside each day to work on that day's math problems. Think of this time as your "math minutes." Working on five problems a day is better than cramming in 20 problems over the weekend.

To prepare properly for class, you'll also need to review vocabulary, understand basic formulas, know how to work cooperatively, and test yourself on your knowledge of the concepts to be covered.

Learn the vocabulary

Like many subjects, math has a specialized vocabulary. If you don't know the most common math terms, you'll have trouble with problems you could otherwise solve. Make a list of key words and study them. Treat math like a foreign language. No one could successfully learn French without studying key vocabulary words in the language. Study math the same way.

Master the formulas

Like math vocabulary, math formulas form the basis for solving math problems. It's important to understand *why* a formula works as it does, but it's also important to know basic formulas so well that you can use them whenever you need them. (See *Tips for memorizing formulas,* page 204.)

Strength in numbers

Traditionally, math hasn't been taught collaboratively. Many instructors have come to realize the benefits of having students study with a partner. Find a willing partner, and work on solving problems together.

Working in collaboration offers many benefits:
• Working with a partner gives you another point of view to consider and will help you to see more possibilities, thus improving your learning.
• Working as a team increases each person's accountability for the material. That accountability includes a responsi-

Advice from the experts

Tips for memorizing formulas

There are many ways to memorize formulas. For instance, you can put them on $3'' \times 5''$ flash cards, color them, and carry them around so you can test yourself anytime. You can also draw the formulas, color them, and put them on a poster to be hung on the wall. You might also consider learning the formulas while listening to music. Play your favorite study music and read a key formula. Then pause, read the formula again, and pause again, letting the music supply the background and serve as a link between the formula on paper and your memory of the formula.

bility to help your colleague understand the material. If you can explain a concept to your partner, you can explain it on a test.

• Offering praise and encouragement to your team member will, in turn, gain you praise and encouragement, thus helping to dispel negative thinking and promote a positive self-image.

Pretest yourself

Don't wait for a scheduled examination to find out how well you know the material. Periodically, give yourself timed tests. Find out what you know — and what you don't know. Most textbooks and several Internet sites offer a wealth of practice questions. Use those questions for your minitest. Check your answers, and review the text

> Okay, but you bring the snacks.

> Let's partner up. We'll be able to get through this math assignment faster and more easily.

whenever you arrive at the wrong answer. You'll thank yourself for these minitests when the real test arrives.

Succeeding on math tests

Math questions generally fall into two categories: number questions or word problems. Although both types involve solving problems and using math principles, several strategies can be used to approach each of these problems.

Number problems

You can count on getting better test scores if you attack number problems correctly. Whether you're taking a standardized test or a teacher-prepared quiz, taking a few simple steps can help you increase your likelihood of success:
• working carefully and deliberately
• writing out all steps
• estimating early
• using all the information in a problem
• reading twice
• being persistent.

Accuracy counts

You'd be amazed how many times students sabotage themselves by approaching math problems in a careless, just-get-it-done kind of way. Careful, deliberate work is required to solve a math problem accurately. (See *Avoiding silly mistakes,* page 206.) To increase your accuracy:
• write carefully
• perform the calculation in reverse, to check your answer
• keep numbers in straight columns
• copy accurately.

Show your work

Remember how you had to show your math work in elementary school? At some point, you probably left that approach to math behind, but showing your work is still good advice. Write out all the steps it takes to solve a problem.

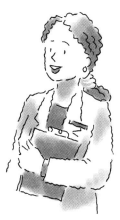

Writing carefully and in columns can increase your accuracy.

You may receive partial credit for a problem even if the final answer isn't correct. In addition, writing out the steps can help you later notice places where you might have gone astray in problems you solve incorrectly.

Estimate early

If you can, estimate each problem's answer before you start to work out the solution. Jot the estimate on a separate sheet, and then solve the problem without thinking about the estimate. When you finish your calculations, compare your answer with the estimate. Are they close?

If not, you might have made a mistake in your calculations, such as missing a decimal point, adding an extra zero, or punching in the wrong number on your calculator. Estimating first helps catch small mistakes that can lead to wrong answers.

Use all the information

Make sure that your calculations use all the information given in the problem. If you think some data is extraneous, double-check it. Few math problems try to trick you by providing too many facts or figures. Most of the time, each piece of information provided is essential in solving the problem.

Read it once, read it twice

After you've found what you hope is the right answer, read the question again. Ask yourself:
• Have I shown my work?
• Did I answer in the correct units?
• Did I answer all parts of the question?
• Does my understanding of the problem on my second reading agree with my understanding after the first reading?

If you answered *yes* to all of the questions, you're probably on the right track.

Don't quit

No matter how effective your approach to solving a problem, you're bound to get stuck here and there. Here are some strategies to employ if you find yourself stuck on a problem:
• Substitute rounded-off numbers for fractions or real numbers for algebraic symbols.
• Pause to think through the problem in its simplest form. Breaking a problem into a simpler form may open up your understanding and allow you solve it in its more complicated form.
• If you have absolutely no idea how to solve a problem, try to figure out what information you're missing. Can you gather clues or missing information in another problem? Can you approximate the information you're missing? Are you really missing something or just not reading the problem well?
• If all else fails, move on to a different question and come back to this problem later.

> If I'm stuck on one of my problems, I take a deep breath and think about the problem in its simplest form.

Word problems

Word problems commonly cause more math anxiety than number problems because the numbers are interwoven with the words. For word problems, there is no substitute for studying well and understanding how to solve specific problems. To make word problems more approachable, you'll need to look at the "big picture," plan well, employ strategies for dealing with difficult word problems, and learn from past mistakes with similar problems.

Exercise your mind

Unlocking tough problems

If you're taking a test and get stuck on an unusually difficult problem, don't waste time trying to solve it the "right way." Imagine yourself trying to open a lock with several keys. Make your best guess about which key — or solution — will fit, and then try it out. If it doesn't work, try another solution. Keep trying various solutions until you find the right "key."

The big picture

When faced with an examination that includes word problems, look the whole test over, skimming the problems and developing a general plan for your work. As you read each problem, jot notes in the margin about how you might go about solving it.

Work on the easiest problems first. They're the ones you can quickly identify the method used for solving the math question. Solving easy problems first will reduce your overall anxiety, foster clear thinking, and get your problem-solving skills warmed up for more difficult problems. It will also help you to earn test points quickly and leave more time to solve more difficult problems.

Watch the clock

Consider planning your time for the whole test as you would plan your time for a study session. Allow more time for problems worth more points. Reserve time at the end of the test to review your work, especially the more difficult problems.

Dealing with the difficult ones

When you're ready to tackle the difficult problems, the first rule is to stay calm. Try not to let the problem overwhelm you. (See *Unlocking tough problems.*) There are several strategies you can use to solve the problem, including:
• marking key words and numbers, which can narrow the problem down to its essential elements
• sketching a diagram of the problem to make the problem more comprehensible

Facing a difficult problem? Take a tip from me: Stay calm!

SNAP

• listing all the formulas you consider relevant to the problem and then deciding with which to begin

• thinking about similar practice problems and how you selected a way to solve them

• guessing at a reasonable answer if the other strategies fail and then checking it. The checking process may suggest a solution method.

Learn from your mistakes

After the test is finished, use it to improve your understanding of the principles involved. After you get a test back from the teacher, read the comments and suggestions. Then, ask yourself:

• Were my errors due to carelessness? For example, did I fail to carry a negative sign from one step to another?

• Did I misread questions? For instance, did I fail to account for all the given data in the solution method?

• Did I consistently miss the same kind of problem?

• Did I remember the formulas incorrectly or incompletely?

• Was I unable to finish the test because I ran out of time?

• Was I unable to solve problems because I hadn't practiced doing similar ones?

• Did I have a difficult time during the test because I was too anxious to focus on the questions?

Based on your answers to these questions, you can identify ways to improve your performance on future tests.

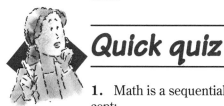

Quick quiz

1. Math is a sequential subject, meaning that every concept:

    A. involves algebra.

    B. builds on a previous concept.

    C. can stand on its own without relating to other concepts.

Answer: B. Because math is a sequential subject, nearly every concept is built on a previous one. That's why skipping assignments can quickly put you behind in your understanding of math as a whole.

2. When taking a math examination filled with word problems, work on the easiest problems:

    A. first.

    B. last.

    C. between more difficult problems.

Answer: A. Solving easy problems first will reduce your anxiety, foster clear thinking, and get your problem-solving skills warmed up for more difficult problems.

3. To handle a problem that provides a number of facts and figures, assume that:

    A. the first facts and figures listed are the most important.

    B. some of the facts and figures were inserted to trick you.

    C. all of the facts and figures are necessary for solving the problem.

Answer: C. Few math problems try to trick you by providing too many facts or figures. Most of the time, each piece of information provided is essential in solving the problem.

Scoring

☆☆☆   If you answered all three questions correctly, stupendous! We've got a math wizard on our hands!

☆☆   If you answered two questions correctly, my, oh, my! And you said you hated math!

☆   If you answered fewer than two questions correctly, don't worry. You're this close to mathematical success!

Using computers to learn

Just the facts

In this chapter, you'll learn:

♦ why the most common computer applications for students include word processing, databases, and telecommunications programs

♦ why most educational software demands only basic computer literacy

♦ how educational software combines a variety of teaching approaches, such as drill and practice, tutorials, and problem solving

♦ how to formulate an effective search, a key to researching on the Internet

♦ how to make the best use of e-mail and electronic mailing lists for research

♦ what online classrooms are and how they can benefit learners.

Computer literacy

Computers play such a prominent role in everyday life that the need to be computer literate is now as basic as the need to read, write, and solve math problems. As you gain computer expertise, you'll become increasingly aware of the value of the electronic world in learning and succeeding in school. Becoming computer literate involves understanding the basics of a computer and software applications. (See *Key computer terminology,* page 212.)

Now I get it!

Key computer terminology

Understanding some key computer-related terms will help you more fully understand how to use a computer and communicate with other computer users.

Main parts

• Hard drive: The hard drive (also known as the C drive in an IBM-compatible computer) is a storage bank for electronic information.

• Memory: Memory is the computer's ability to store and process information. Computers with large amounts of memory can operate more applications and store more files than computers with less memory.

• Modem: A modem enables a computer to transmit data over telephone lines. For home computers, the modem allows the computer to connect to the Internet and use e-mail.

• Monitor: Also known as the display screen, the monitor shows the text and graphics displayed by the computer.

• Mouse: The mouse moves a cursor around the monitor and allows the user to point to an object, open files and folders, and perform nearly all other functions of a computer.

• RAM: The amount of random-access memory (RAM) in a computer is an indication of the speed at which the computer can operate. For instance, a computer with 32 megabytes (MB) of RAM can operate considerably faster than a computer with 16 MB of RAM.

Outside the computer

• CD-ROM: A CD-ROM, which stands for compact disk, read-only memory, is a circular plastic disk that can hold a great deal of information in electronic form. Most CD-ROMs can hold 64 MB of information, more than 44 times what a standard 3½" diskette can hold.

• Diskette: Also called a floppy, a diskette is a rigid, portable device for carrying electronic information. Diskettes, each 3½" wide, can hold 1.44 MB of information in electronic form.

• Network: A network is a group of two or more computers linked together. Businesses and universities often use networks to allow computers to share information easily.

• Printer: A printer is used to display text or illustrations on paper. Numerous types of printer are available, including laser and ink-jet printers. Many printers use black ink only, but some use colored ink and, therefore, are capable of printing colored text or photos.

• Scanner: A scanner reads texts or illustrations on paper and translates the information into a form the computer can use. The text or graphics can then be manipulated on the computer.

I may not be a computer guru, but understanding the language helps me navigate the world of computers.

Computer basics

To understand how to use a computer, you need first to understand the difference between hardware and software and the major components of each.

Software vs. hardware

Software refers to the written instructions that tell a computer how to operate. Software tells the computer how to begin running, for example. Word processing programs, database programs, and E-mail programs are types of software.

Hardware refers to the electronic equipment that carries out software instructions. The central processing unit (CPU) is the brain of the computer and consists of the arithmetic-logic unit, the control unit, and memory — devices that work together to drive all computer operations. The big box you've probably seen under or beside a monitor houses the CPU.

Other hardware devices include storage devices, such as the floppy disk drive and the CD-ROM drive, display devices such as the monitor, input devices such as the keyboard and mouse, and output devices such as a printer.

Interface

Most computers and student-oriented software programs are user-friendly, which means they have a simple-to-use interface. The term *interface* refers to the way the user interacts with the software. For instance, typical word processing programs use a group of menus across the top of the screen to carry out particular functions. Each menu — such as File, Edit, View, Insert, Format, Tools, Table, Window, Help, and others — can carry out certain commands. The user selects the menu by clicking on it, then selects the desired menu command from a list of possible commands.

This menu function is part of the interface, as are command symbols called icons, rulers, dialog boxes (that pop up at certain times during the operation of a program to tell the user what can be done or alert the user to a problem), and numerous other functions.

The easier a program is to operate, the more user-friendly its interface is said to be. Today most software programs, or applications, nearly run themselves. Their interfaces are so well defined that they can lead the user

Advice from the experts

Help!

Most software applications contain help menus to assist you in operating the program. The help feature is usually listed as a menu option or marked by a question mark symbol (?). Help menus usually list basic steps for operating the program as well as more advanced hints and shortcuts. The illustration shows a table of contents for a typical help menu.

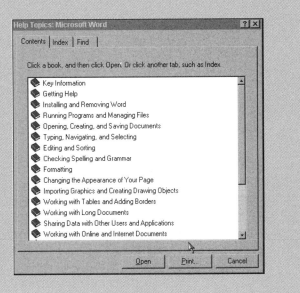

through programs step-by-step and offer clear, simply written instructions for answering questions and troubleshooting problems. (See *Help!*)

Desktops vs. laptops

Most personal computers sold today are desktop systems, which typically consist of a full-sized monitor, keyboard, mouse, speakers, and a CPU. Laptops, also known as notebooks, are smaller, easily portable computers that can run from an electrical outlet or from battery power.

IBM-compatible vs. Macintosh

Most personal computers sold in the United States are IBM-compatible, meaning they use the same operating language as early personal computers developed by International Business Machines (IBM) in the late 1980s. Other personal computers sold in this country are Macintosh-compatible, meaning that they use the same operating language as Macintosh computers, produced chiefly by Apple Computers, Inc.

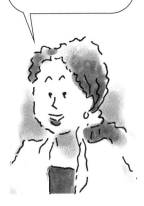

With today's user-friendly programs, a single click of the mouse provides all the help you need to run a program.

Both types of personal computers are capable of performing the same functions in just about all software applications available today. The decision of whether to use or buy an IBM-compatible or Macintosh-compatible computer is a matter of personal taste more than a matter of either computer's capabilities.

Common applications

Legions of software applications have been — and continue to be — developed for just about every possible use. For students, the most important types of software applications to be familiar with include:
- word processors
- database programs
- spreadsheet programs
- graphics and other design applications.

When it's all about the words

Word processors are software applications designed primarily to create, edit, store, and print textual material. These programs have made the typewriter nearly obsolete because they handle text more flexibly than a typewriter ever could.

Word processors encourage students to become better writers by enabling them to revise their work quickly and easily. Most word processing programs can check spelling and grammar to help eliminate errors. (See *Spellchecking software,* page 216.) Common word processing programs include Microsoft Word, WordPerfect, and Apple Works.

When it's all about the data

Database programs store and organize large amounts of data electronically. Databases are used by individuals, public agencies, and businesses to store and retrieve large amounts of information quickly and easily.

To understand how a database works, imagine that the database is a huge post office with hundreds, thousands, tens of thousands, even millions of individual mailboxes on the wall. Each mailbox is numbered and can contain any kind of electronic information you'd like to store in it, from a single word or number to an entire file of words or numbers to whole groups of files.

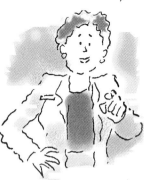

Use word processing software when you want to handle text quickly and easily.

Advice from the experts

Spellchecking software

Spellchecking software works by matching every word in the text against an internal dictionary. If the computer can't find a match for a word, it flags the word for you to verify. A flagged word doesn't mean the word is spelled incorrectly; it just means that the spellchecker's dictionary doesn't contain that particular word.

Check it once
Be aware that spellchecking software won't catch nonspelling errors in your paper. For example, a spellchecker catches misspelled words but can't catch misused words. If you type *their* instead of *there* or *they're*, or *them* instead of *then*, the spellchecker won't flag the errors because the words you've mistakenly used are valid words.

Check it twice
A spellchecker will also overlook times when you've omitted a word as well as made other grammatical mistakes. Some grammatical mistakes can be found using a grammar checker, and some spellcheckers contain a basic grammar checker to spot instances of repeated words and other simple errors. However, no spellchecker or grammar checker can catch all mistakes. Use of these software applications demands your attention to make sure all mistakes are found.

The database allows you to retrieve certain kinds of information in a particular sequence. For instance, you can request a database filled with names and addresses to give you an alphabetical listing of everyone whose last name begins with J, M, S, and V and to provide you with each person's first name, followed by the last name, followed by the words, "my friend," followed by the person's address. In a flash, that's what the database will display.

Information within a database can be added, deleted, and updated quickly and easily so the user is assured of having the most current information available. Students can find many applications for a database, particularly for compiling research materials and notes. Commonly used database programs include Microsoft Access and Filemaker Pro.

When it's all about the numbers

A spreadsheet is basically an electronic ledger with vertical columns and horizontal rows for holding and tabulating numeric data. The user creates the format of the spreadsheet, enters the formulas necessary to compute the data, and enters the data into appropriate locations, or cells, within the spreadsheet. The computer then calculates the data automatically and displays the results.

Businesses find that current and accurate data in spreadsheets can serve as the basis for making well-informed financial decisions. Students can make use of spreadsheet software to help them in mathematics, laboratory science, social studies, business management, and numerous other courses. Common spreadsheet programs include Apple Works and Microsoft Excel.

When it's all about the images

With graphics software, the user can create a variety of visual images. Graphics software applications typically allow the user to create illustrations using preformatted shapes or a freehand drawing implement. The computer artist can change the image by enlarging or reducing it, changing colors, rotating it, animating it, or performing a host of other functions to create the precise image desired. Commonly used graphic software applications include Adobe Photoshop, Adobe Illustrator, Microsoft Paint, and Macromedia Freehand.

Telecommunications

Telecommunications is the process of sending and receiving data by electronic means. E-mail and the Internet both make use of telecommunications technology.

E-mail

The term *e-mail,* which stands for electronic mail, refers to the ability to send a written message from one computer to another. Through e-mail, users can send letters, memos, and other information to other computer users anywhere in the world. Microsoft Outlook Express and Eudora are popular e-mail programs.

Internet

The Internet is an enormously complex system of linked computers that gives users throughout the world access to information and the ability to conduct business over telephone or cable lines. The World Wide Web (WWW) — or Web, for short — is a huge part of the Internet. More and more businesses today are using the Web to promote their services or sell their products. Students use the Web to tap into untold numbers of resources they normally wouldn't be able to obtain. Microsoft Internet Explorer and Netscape Navigator are popular Internet-access programs, or browsers.

Computer-assisted instruction

Learning by computer, or computer-assisted instruction (CAI), has become popular in the last few years to help fulfill a variety of educational goals. The most effective CAI programs require only basic computer skills. Many CAI applications combine a variety of formats to offer the student various ways to learn. Common CAI formats include:
- drill and practice
- tutorial
- simulation
- computer-managed instruction
- problem solving.

Repeat and improve

Drill-and-practice software allows learners to master facts, relationships, problems, and vocabulary. The software usually offers groups of questions having similar content, which allows the student to hone specific skills. The software may be designed to offer more difficult questions as the student progresses through the application.

Tutor-in-a-box

Tutorial software aims to teach concepts rather than allow the practice of individual skills. This software presents concepts in a number of formats, including text and images, and commonly incorporates feedback to student responses. Tutorials may employ pretesting or posttesting to instruct students at the appropriate teaching level.

Simulated scenarios

A simulation is a computer-generated visual and auditory experience. Computer simulations allow students to experience real-life events in the safety of the classroom. Because simulations usually demand decision-making skills, the student becomes directly involved in the outcomes.

Computer-assisted instruction can be a boon to students with families and full-time jobs.

Management by computer

Computer-managed instruction assesses the knowledge level and educational goals of students. Through computerized testing, this software can help instructors assess students and design a curriculum to fit their needs.

Solving problems

Problem-solving software is useful after a student is familiar with basic necessary concepts. Problem-solving software can then help students use their concepts to solve difficult problems and advance their level of thinking.

Learning online

Use of the Internet, particularly the Web and E-mail, has been increasing at a staggering rate. People use the Internet for business, entertainment, correspondence, and hundreds of other uses, including research and attending online classrooms.

Online research

The Web is based on the ability to link one document to another through the use of hyperlinks, which typically appear on screen as buttons, graphics, or blue, underlined words. Clicking a hyperlink sends the user to another document, which commonly also contains hyperlinks, which can send the user to still more documents. Moving from document to document — or pages, as they're called — is termed *surfing the Web*.

A Web page may contain text, hyperlinks, or graphics in any combination. A single Web site may contain just two or three pages or hundreds of pages organized according to the type of information they contain. The main page for each site is called the home page; all other pages branch off this page. Understanding how sites are named, how to find the site you're looking for, and how to gauge the reliability of the information you find are all important in getting the most from online research.

Is this what they mean by surfing the Web? Wheeeeee!

Site names

In the United States, Web sites are categorized according to whether they're owned by a business, an individual, an educational institution, or a government agency. Each site owner is assigned a particular suffix to its Web site name, each suffix coming after a period:

• com, for *commercial.* Addresses ending in *.com* (commonly pronounced *dot com*) are typically reserved for individuals and businesses.

• edu, for *educational.* Addresses ending in *.edu* (commonly pronounced *dot e-d-u*) are reserved for educational institutions, such as colleges and universities.

• gov, for *governmental.* Addresses ending in *.gov* (commonly pronounced *dot guv*) are reserved for government institutions and agencies.

• net, for network. Addresses ending in *.net* (commonly pronounced *dot net*) are generally reserved for Internet service providers.

• org, for *organization.* Addresses ending in *.org* (commonly pronounced *dot org*) are reserved for nonprofit organizations and associations.

Addresses

Every page on the Web has its own address, called a universal resource locator, or URL. Most URLs begin with *http://,* an acronym for hypertext transfer protocol. This abbreviation is typically (but not always) followed by *www.,* followed by each particular page's address. For example, a home page for a company named "Marvin Acme Produce" might have *http://www.marvinacmeproduce.com* as its home page address. A related page listing the types of fruits offered by the company might be named *http://www.marvinacmeproduce.com/index/fruits/htm.*

Search engines

With millions and millions of pages on the Web, finding the information a particular user is looking for has become increasingly difficult. Imagine walking into a library with tens of millions of books and articles, thousands of which relate in some way to the particular topic you're looking for. How do you sort through all those sources quickly and easily?

On the Web, you'll use a search engine. Search engines allow Web users to enter keywords to find the information they want. For instance, if you enter a keyword such as "diabetes education" into the Search box of a search engine, the engine will try to find all the pages it thinks you might be looking for and then supply a list of those pages and a hypertext link so you can go from the search page to the page you're looking for.

How they work

Today's search engines use complicated formulas to figure out what kind of information a user is trying to find. For example, the search engine might count the number of times *diabetes education* occurs as a unit on a page, the number of times the words occur in isolation, and the number of times either word is used on the page. It then calculates the likelihood of that page meeting your needs, and then lists all the pages it finds, starting with the ones it thinks you're most likely to want. No search engine can provide exactly the sites you're looking for, of course, so if you can't find what you're looking for using one search engine, try another one. (See *Smart searching,* page 222.)

Marking your favorite pages

Web browsers contain a page-marking feature that allows you to mark sites you enjoy visiting or, for whatever reason, think you'll visit again. Think of it as folding over the corner of a page in a favorite book so you can return quickly to that page. Bookmarking favorite Web pages cuts the amount of time required to find that site again the next time you visit the Web.

Reliability of Web resources

After you've located a document that seems to supply the information you're looking for, you'll need to judge the reliability of the content. The phrase, "Don't believe everything you read," takes on renewed importance with the Internet. It's vital that you compare sources to verify information and be alert to sources you've never heard of that contain information of questionable validity or provide seemingly reliable information in a way that makes it seem as if they're pushing their own biased agenda.

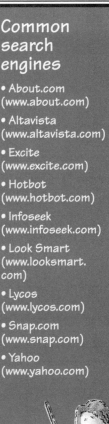

Common search engines

- About.com (www.about.com)
- Altavista (www.altavista.com)
- Excite (www.excite.com)
- Hotbot (www.hotbot.com)
- Infoseek (www.infoseek.com)
- Look Smart (www.looksmart.com)
- Lycos (www.lycos.com)
- Snap.com (www.snap.com)
- Yahoo (www.yahoo.com)

Advice from the experts

Smart searching

Conducting an Internet search is getting easier and easier as search engines refine the way they look for Web pages. Try these tips for getting the most out of your Internet searches:

Forming a search

• Be aware that most search engines pay no attention at all to such words as *the, a, an,* or to plural forms of keywords. You can save time by omitting these words from your search.

• Most searches aren't case sensitive, meaning that uppercase letters don't matter. Save time and effort by typing everything in lowercase.

• Most search engines treat text found between two sets of quotation marks as a unit. If you're looking for information about the famed neuropsychologist Benjamin Bloom, try searching for "benjamin bloom" with quotes surrounding his name.

• Try not to use too broad a term as your keyword. For instance, a search for the keyword *diabetes* could return a list containing thousands of documents. A more narrow search for *diabetes education* or *diabetes treatment* will help your search engine return pages more likely to meet your needs.

• Don't make your keywords too specific. For example, a search for the keywords *diabetes education in Kentucky during the Eisenhower era* might return no results at all. A search for *diabetes education and Eisenhower,* however, might be broad enough to pull the documents you're looking for.

If at first you don't succeed

• If your first search doesn't return what you're looking for, try rephrasing your keywords to be more inclusive or less inclusive. Try using different words. Think of the search engine as a huge index. Normally when you go to an index and can't find what you're looking for, you look for related terms or phrases. Do the same thing when conducting an Internet search.

• If you've rephrased your keywords and the search is still coming up short, try another search engine. You'd be amazed how many times a search in one search engine comes up with hardly any information at all, and the identical search in another search engine comes up with precisely what you need.

• Know that most search engines offer advanced searching capabilities that allow you to select from a range of options to narrow your search more precisely. Check for an Advanced Search button when your search bogs down without providing you with the information you need.

As a general rule, information contained in the pages of government agencies, main university sites (not sites belonging to individual students within a university), and sites of businesses or agencies known to be of good repute tend to be reliable. (See *Great starter sites,* page 224.) Information contained in an individual's site or the site of a small, unknown organization or foundation tends to be less reliable. To be safe, always treat whatever information you find on the Web with a critical eye.

E-mail and electronic mailing lists

Students can also find information through the use of e-mail and electronic mailing lists. Both require Internet access, but neither is difficult to understand or to master. If you don't have Internet access at home or work, try your school or local library.

E-mail

E-mail is a rapid form of written communication between individuals with access to the Internet. When you gain access to the Internet, you'll receive an e-mail address, typically a user-defined set of letters or numbers, always followed by the symbol @ and then by the Internet service provider's address. For instance, an e-mail address for Suzanne Jones might be *sjones54@hotmail.com*.

With e-mail access comes the ability to send and receive messages, including files that might be attached to a message. Most of the time, a message sent from any computer anywhere in the world reaches its destination within about 5 minutes from the time it was sent. However, longer delays commonly occur, and some messages never reach their destination.

Researching with e-mail

E-mail offers students several ways to find information. For instance, many sites include e-mail addresses and encourage comments and questions. If you're willing to wait for a response, many organizations and universities can prove helpful in providing information in response to an e-mail. In addition, e-mail can be used to correspond easily with researchers anywhere in the world. Many researchers prefer corresponding over e-mail than over the telephone because they can correspond by e-mail at their convenience.

Electronic mailing lists

An electronic mailing list is a list of e-mail addresses organized around a particular area of interest. For instance, you can sign up on a publisher's electronic mailing list that will automatically e-mail information about new books relating to cancer or on a museum's electronic mailing list that e-mails information about the newest exhibit arriving next week. Some electronic mailing lists allow online discussions about particular topics.

Advice from the experts

Great starter sites

Everyone new to the Internet needs to start somewhere. Here are addresses and owners of some health care sites to get you started. Type the address exactly as it appears here in the Address bar of your Web browser, and hit the Enter key. Enjoy!

Owner	Address	Related facts
American Nurses Association	*www.nursingworld.org*	Professional nursing association; offers news about current nursing issues, information on fellowship programs, and online journals
Healthway Online	*www.healthanswers.com*	Offers an online newsletter, news about current health issues, a searchable drug database, and reference material
Lippincott Williams & Wilkins	*www.nursingcenter.com*	Publisher of *Lippincott Manual of Nursing Practice* and other nursing and health care books and journals; offers health care news, continuing education credits, journal archives, and e-mail accounts
Mayo Health Center	*www.mayohealth.org*	Publishes the *Mayo Clinic Health Letter;* offers a searchable library of health-related information for patients and health care providers
National Institutes of Health (NIH)	*www.nih.gov*	Main site for all NIH sites, including the National Heart, Lung, and Blood Institute, National Cancer Institute, National Institute of Child Health and Development, and others
Nurses Service Organization	*www.nso.com*	Insurance products for health care professionals; offers policy information and monthly case studies
Springhouse Corporation	*www.springnet.com*	Publisher of *Nursing2000* and other nursing and health care books and journals; offers continuing education credits, NCLEX-RN preparatory services, journal archives, conference listings, employment guidance, and numerous links
WellnessWeb	*www.wellweb.com*	Independent site; offers basic information for patients about a variety of common diseases, and numerous links to research articles

Electronic mailing lists are generally controlled by a manager who weeds out bizarre or offensive postings. Many professionals belong to electronic mailing lists relevant to their fields. To find out which electronic mailing lists you might make effective use of, ask your instructors or upper-level students what electronic mailing lists they've joined.

Online classrooms

Online classrooms offer presentations on specific topics, question-and-answer sessions and, in some cases, assignments from an instructor with resulting feedback. The Internet service provider America Online offers free online courses on many topics. Other fee-for-service online classrooms, many associated with colleges and universities, are growing in popularity.

Courses offered online typically cost less than the same course taught the traditional way, a benefit for students on a tight budget. The courses also usually require the same kinds of assignments as those assigned in traditional classes. Tests can be sent and returned by e-mail or downloaded (saved on the user's hard drive) from the sponsor's Web site.

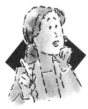

Quick quiz

1. A database is a software application that allows you to:
   A. tabulate numeric data easily.
   B. create or edit graphic images.
   C. retrieve information in a particular sequence.
Answer: C. A database allows you to retrieve certain kinds of information in a particular sequence.

2. If you saw the address *marvinacme@worldnet.att.net,* you'd know the address was:
   A. an e-mail account.
   B. a newsgroup.
   C. a Web page.
Answer: A. The @ symbol in an address means it's an e-mail address. Web addresses and newsgroups don't contain the @ symbol.

3. An electronic mailing list is:
   A. an Internet discussion group that occurs in real time.
   B. a list of e-mail addresses organized around a particular topic.
   C. a list of topics found at a Web site.

Answer: B. An electronic mailing list is organized by topic and is commonly used by students and professionals in a particular field.

Scoring

☆☆☆   If you answered all three questions correctly, tremendous! You're technologically savvy and suited for cyber-learning!

☆☆   If you answered two questions correctly, super! You're ready to apply yourself to some software applications!

☆   If you answered fewer than two questions correctly, keep cybercool. You'll be @ upper URL levels soon enough!

Glossary and index

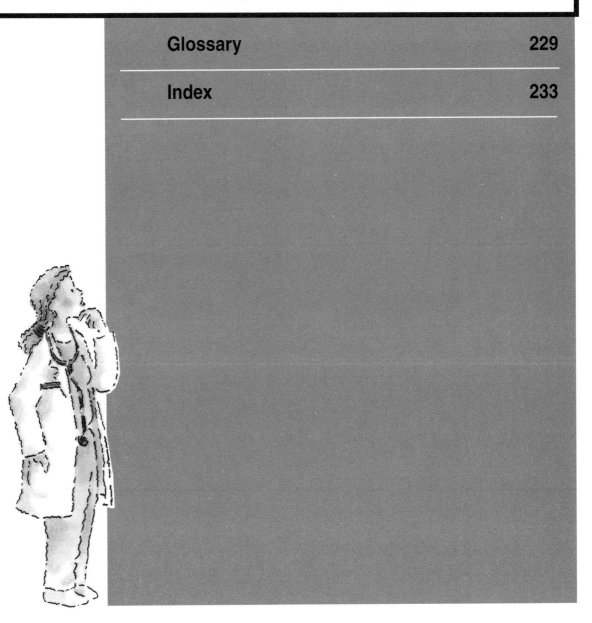

Glossary

Acronym: word created from the first letter or letters of each part or major parts of a compound term; used as a memory aid

Acrostic: word or phrase created from the first letter of each item in a list; used as a memory aid

Active listening: using planned strategies, such as taking notes or asking questions, to remember important concepts and supporting details

Active reading: anticipating ideas and reading for a purpose; continually posing questions and searching for answers; used to gain a full understanding of the author's message

Affirmations: repetitious, positive self-talk that usually involves simple phrases about one's capabilities

Anxiety: general uneasiness, apprehension, or worry

Association: process of remembering one item because of its connection to another item; linking ideas to facilitate learning

Attitude: how a person approaches a task or situation; involves thoughts, feelings and behavior

Attractive distracters: incorrect options on multiple-choice tests; considered attractive because they may seem correct

Background: part of a research paper that gives a history of the topic; may also introduce other areas of the topic or explain new terminology

Behavior modification: type of external motivation involving rewards; used to divert focus from the dread of a task

Bias: favoring one side of an issue; expressing personal opinion

Bibliography: list of sources relevant to a topic and worth consideration with title, author, and date of publication in each entry

Biographical indices: information about the lives of important people, usually including personal and professional information

Bloom's taxonomy: system developed in 1956 by Benjamin S. Bloom to describe seven levels of understanding

Blue book: blue-covered booklets often used for written examinations

Brain waves: indication of biochemical activity in the brain involving the transmission of electrical impulses with the type of wave depending on the state of mind — for example, alpha when alert and relaxed, beta when wide awake and active, delta when sound asleep, and theta when near sleep

Burnout: state that results from working too long without breaks with signs that include fatigue, boredom, and stress

Chapter map: visual arrangement used to explain relationships among concepts and an author's patterns of thought

Classification systems: how libraries code their holdings using letter and number combinations called *call numbers;* for example, Dewey Decimal System or Library of Congress System

Closure: positive feeling that comes from completing a task, as opposed to the anxious feeling that may result from unfinished business

Combination test: test that contains more than one type of question; for example, essay, multiple-choice, short-answer, or true-false questions

Comprehension: understanding; using skills that include concentration, decoding, and association

Comprehensive examination: examination, usually written, that tests mastery of an entire field or curriculum; test that covers all material presented since the beginning of a term

Computer-assisted instruction: use of computers for instructional tasks, such as drills and practice tests

Computer simulation: program that allows students to experience real-life events in the safety of a classroom

Concentration: focus; ignoring distractions that may impair study habits or quality of work

Conclusion: last part of a research paper that restates the thesis, briefly summarizes key points, and usually ends with a succinct, moving statement

Cortex: part of the brain responsible for most high-level functions, such as sight and coordination

Counterargument and rebuttal: part of a research paper that states opposing viewpoints and assesses their strengths and weaknesses

Cramming: an unproductive study method in which a person frantically tries to memorize a lot of information in a short period of time

Critical thinking: recalling prior knowledge to translate, interpret, process, and apply new information

Database: vast amounts of data organized for rapid search and retrieval (as by a computer)

Esteem: assurance that one is accepted and valued; usually referring to self-esteem

Flash card: card with a term or question on one side and the definition or answer on the other side; common study aid

General adaptation syndrome: theory by Hans Selye that defines the body's reaction to stress as a syndrome evolving in three stages: alarm, resistance, and exhaustion

Goal: End toward which effort is directed; short-term or long-term aim relating to specific, measurable outcomes

Goal structure: how students relate to others who are also working toward goals; categorized as cooperative, competitive, or individualistic

Graphic: illustration or visual image

Hardware: equipment; electronic computer components that carry out software instructions

Hook: memory aid, such as a picture, pattern, rhyme, or story (*see* Association)

Idea map (mind or concept map): visual representation to show how information relates that usually presents central ideas and peripheral facts as a tree and its branches

Introduction: first part of a research paper, which may include a statement of the problem, related literature review, conceptual or theoretical framework, purpose of the paper, and definitions of key terms

Journaling: keeping a personal journal; recording events, thoughts, and feelings

Learning: incorporating new information; gaining knowledge; changing behavior

Learning process: receiving information, gradually understanding the information, assimilating the information, and making it useful

Local-area network (LAN): linked computers geographically close together, usually in the same building

Long-term memory: ability of the brain to remember information for long periods, the duration of which directly relates to the meaningfulness of the memory; also called semantic memory

Main body: central part of a research paper, which uses logical organization to explain ideas

Management plan: tool used to organize and prioritize tasks and goals

Mantra: syllable, word, or phrase repeated again and again; used in the technique of transcendental meditation

Memory[1]: retention and processing of information that involves registration, working memory, short-term memory, and long-term memory; lowest level of understanding in Bloom's taxonomy

Memory[2]: where the computer stores information, on the hard drive or a disk

Mental pictures: most common way for the mind to process information; often called *the key to memorizing*

Mnemonics: memory aids, such as *acronyms, acrostics, associations,* and rhymes

Mnemonigraph: memory aid that involves drawing or diagramming information

Motivation: reason for doing something, which can be internal or external

Network: interrelated group or system; two or more linked computer systems

Neurons: nerve cells; structures that transmit messages to, from, and within the brain

Newsgroups: electronic bulletin boards comprised of e-mail messages to which users need not subscribe and can respond individually to any posted message

Noncomprehensive examination: test that covers information presented only since the last test

Objective test: examination that involves choosing among provided answers; for example, multiple-choice, matching, or true-false questions

Objectivity: ability to report information without personal opinion or bias

Open-book examination: examination in which the student is allowed to use supplementary materials, such as notes, textbooks, charts, or crib sheets; tests a student's ability to locate and process information quickly

Optical scanner: device that can read text or illustrations printed on paper and translate the information into a format a computer can use

Oral examination: examination used to measure a student's ability to analyze and integrate information as well as the ability to respond quickly in an organized manner; often given as a final test before awarding a degree

Outlining: sequential process of organizing information according to major concepts and supporting details

Overlearning: reviewing the same information several times using different study methods

Overstudy: continuing to study after the point at which the material is known

P-A-G-E: acronym for *prepare, ask, gather, evaluate;* multilayered study process that is more effective than reading and highlighting only

Paraphrase: restate main ideas and explanations rather than memorizing material word-for-word

Parasympathetic nervous system: part of the nervous system responsible for slowing vital signs and causing relaxation of smooth muscle and sphincters

Passive note-taking: using taped or borrowed notes

Plagiarism: using another person's work without citing the source; treated as stealing

Postlecture reading: additional resources not covered during class that help a student focus on information emphasized in a lecture and deepen a student's understanding of the subject

Practice: repetition that may involve silent rereading, rewriting, diagramming, vocalizing, or discussing information

Prepared cramming: pretest review session done by a student who has been studying wisely

Pretest: use of a test to evaluate baseline knowledge at a point before another test with similar content

Previewing: recalling previous knowledge of a subject to create a mental outline of upcoming class information

Primary sources: original documents, such as speeches or books, used in research

Procrastination: putting off activities until later; letting low-priority tasks get in the way of high-priority ones

Progressive relaxation: technique of gradually releasing control of each muscle from head to toe

Reciprocal teaching: technique for practicing reading comprehension that involves the use of five strategies good readers use most when reading: prediction, clarification, visualization, questioning, and summarizing

Recitation: orally replying to study questions; useful study technique sometimes used as a classroom exercise

Registration: receiving and acknowledging new information without understanding it

Regressing: constantly rereading; a habit that slows reading speed

Rehearsal: repetition that may involve spaced study, previewing, recitation, study partners, or overlearning

Rehearsal process: reading material, thinking about it, reciting it, answering questions and then repeating the process

Reserved books: books temporarily removed from a library, usually at the request of faculty member, to be used by students in a particular class

Rough draft: first writing effort; putting ideas on paper in any order

Schedule: time-management tool that can be long-term or short-term and should include study time

Secondary sources: documents that interpret, evaluate, describe, or otherwise restate the work of primary sources

Serotonin: chemical in the brain that can strongly affect mood and emotion

Short-term memory: ability of the brain to store information briefly, which lasts only seconds or minutes unless reinforced; also called episodic memory

Skimming: first phase of reading that involves looking at pictures, captions, headings, introductory paragraphs, and table of contents; often called previewing

Social network: relationships among people in a group

Social support: people who provide assistance in meeting basic needs

Software: written instructions, or programs, that tell a computer how to operate

Spaced study: alternating study sessions with breaks; very beneficial when alternating fifteen minutes of study with very short breaks; also known as distributed practice

Spreadsheet: ledger with vertical columns and horizontal rows, usually used for numerical data; computer accounting program

SQ3R: acronym for survey, question, read, recite, and review; a classic study system

Stress: the body's response to demands, which appears as worry, concern, anxiety, or nervousness and can be beneficial (eustress) or damaging (distress)

Stressor: source of stress that can be almost any stimulus but commonly involves a conflict

Subjective test: test that requires unique answers and is used to measure recall of information and skills in organizing and expressing ideas and may include short-answer, essay, or fill-in-the-blank questions

Take-home examination: essentially an open-book examination but with more time allowed; usually more difficult than in-class examinations

Telecommunication: sending and receiving data by electronic means

Test anxiety: test-taking situation that causes a student to experience a mental block, which may happen even if the student knows the material well

Text labeling: note-taking while reading that involves identifying relationships and summarizing information; creating a kind of index to locate information more quickly

Text marking: highlighting, underlining, or otherwise marking the text while reading; taking notes in the margin

Text structure: how the vocabulary and topics of a text are organized

Thesaurus: resource that provides synonyms, antonyms, slang terms, and related words for each entry

Thesis statement: purpose of a paper; a single, complete, declarative sentence in which major assertions or conclusions are written

Time management: means of controlling and organizing a schedule for maximum efficiency

Time planning: looking ahead to organize a schedule that may refer to 1 semester, 1 week, or 1 day

To-do list: listing of immediate goals placed in order of priority

Trigger words: words that provide keys to an author's message; easy-to-spot, repeatedly used terms that present themes, vocabulary, or central ideas

Understanding: ability to make important connections among ideas; relating new information to existing knowledge

Visual aids: elements, such as maps, charts, diagrams, photographs, and illustrations, that are used to explain ideas

Visualization: use of mental imagery to link objects or ideas, which may involve imagining a new solution to a problem

Wide-area network (WAN): computers linked usually by telephone lines or radio waves over a distance

Withdrawal: physical or psychological retreat; usually resulting from anxiety or fear; social or emotional detachment

Word map: study aid used to remember vocabulary terms that involves grouping words according to general headings

Working memory: ability of the brain to select, associate, organize, and rehearse information

Index

i refers to an illustration; t refers to a table.

i refers to an illustration; t refers to a table.

i refers to an illustration; t refers to a table.

i refers to an illustration; t refers to a table.

i refers to an illustration; t refers to a table.

Notes

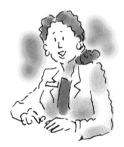

Notes

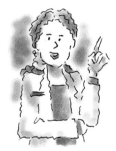

Notes

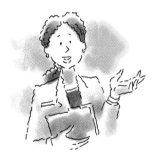

Notes

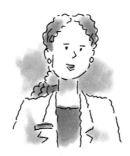

Notes

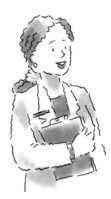

Notes

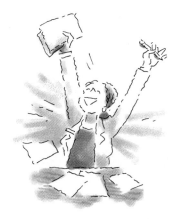

Notes

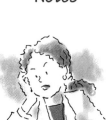